Performance diagnosis and purchase examination of elite sport horses

Performance diagnosis and purchase examination of elite sport horses

CESMAS 2010

edited by:

Arno Lindner

Arbeitsgruppe Pferd

Wageningen Academic
Publishers

ISBN: 978-90-8686-147-7
e-ISBN: 978-90-8686-701-1
DOI: 10.3920/978-90-8686-701-1

Cover photo: Geir Rom Haugerud, Norway
Photos inside cover: Marianne Sloet,
Geir Haugerud and Arno Lindner

First published, 2010

Foreword

CESMAS, and the idea behind it, is 14 years old. In 1996 it was decided to have every 2 years in Europe a meeting focussing on the Sport Horse. Since then CESMAS has been held in Córdoba (1998), Taormina/Messina (2000), Saumur (2002), Oslo (2004), Cambridge (2006), Utrecht (2008) and now in Sigtuna! The meetings were always in one of the countries where one of the European committee members originated from, in most cases even in the hometown. With this meeting we are 'through': CESMAS has been hosted by each European committee member once in her/his home.

What now? This question does not have a clear answer at this moment. Several options are available: (1) We stop it. Easiest option! We get older and have or may have other interests. (2) We can run it in North America. Two committee members live in the USA and we have discussed this option several times. However, it is not easy to realize. There are many reasons that in the sum produce a very high hurdle to be overcome. Let me mention two of them: the currency conversion and the tax policy. (3) Me running it at a 'preferred' place in Europe. Everything started in 1996 in Bonn with the annual meeting of the Association for Equine Sports Medicine. A CESMAS in Germany has not been held. (4) A new format is used. This because the original idea is still valid as there is no international conference focussing on Sport Horses. However, the time and money to be spend in meetings has not increased, but the number of yearly conferences is much higher than back in the 1990ties and there are lots more of speciality events, that professionals need to follow to obtain or maintain their accreditations. Can CESMAS compete?

We will know in 2 years time!

CESMAS 2010 will deal with 'Performance diagnosis and purchase examination of elite sport horses'. It was decided to present most of the subjects on this theme as complex as they are. Thus, two, sometimes several more, experts in the respective field were asked to cooperate to integrate the information. This is not easy for professionals making a daily living and in some instance not knowing well or at all each other. The results are here in the book. I am very grateful for their effort and like the result! Thank you very much! It has been a pleasure to work with you!

A pleasure will be also to hold the meeting in Sigtuna, the hometown of Arne Lindholm. Would you have known that there it is so pretty Arne would have had much more competition than he already has! Thank you very much Arne, for being willing to do it!

And finally, thank you members of the scientific committee for all the help to prepare this meeting! I enjoyed thoroughly all the discussions and meetings and will miss them in the case that we stop to run CESMAS. Everything keeps changing!

I would like to wish readers pleasure reading the book.

Arno

Scientific Committee

Warwick M. Bayly, USA
Hilary Clayton, USA
Anne Courroucé-Malblanc, France
Sue Dyson, United Kingdom
Adriana Ferlazzo, Italy
Arne Holm, Norway
Arne Lindholm, Sweden
Arno Lindner, Germany
José Luis López Rivero, Spain
Marianne Sloet van Oldruitenborgh-Oosterbaan, the Netherlands

Table of contents

Can genetics help to find THE horse; positive and negative markers of performance and health

Eric Barrey
Integrative Biology and Exercise Adaptation U902, INSERM, Genopole Evry, France
Animal Genetics and Integrative Biology UMR 1313, INRA Jouy-en-Josas, France

Introduction

With the rapid progress in equine genetics, new applications in early performance evaluation and health markers detection become available. With the great development of biotechnologies, many new biomolecular tools will change the way to manage the horse selection and disease diagnostic and treatment. The recent equine genome sequencing by an international consortium (Wade *et al.*, 2009) was the major genetic result that will impact in the near future all the other equine genomics. The purpose of this article is to give an overview of the new developments in equine genomics for performance evaluation and health markers after a short summary of the previous knowledge about the genetic components of the exercise performance traits.

Genetic component of the performance traits: how to measure the heritability estimates?

With the development of equine science, more functional traits can be measured for early evaluation of exercise ability. The objective is to predict the level of performance that a young horse can reach by measuring some physiological characteristics during an exercise test. For a breeding purpose, the heritability of each trait should be determined to know if it is useful for breeding selection. This article presents the heritability estimates of some locomotor and physiological traits related to the equine exercise ability. Several exercise traits have been studied in different breeds: muscle fibre types, heart rate, blood lactate, gaits, jump style and morphology.

Methods

Heritability estimates (h^2) of the exercise traits have been calculated in order to estimate the influence of genetic and environment components. Heritability is the ratio between genetic variance and the total variance including environmental effects. For each variable, the variance components are calculated using Restricted Maximum Likelihood Resolution (REML). The genetic variance is estimated by the following variance analysis model including fixed and random effects. The relationship between all effects are taken into account for the random Animal effect:

$$Y_{ijklmn} = Age_i + Height_{ij} + Track_{ijk} + Breed_{ijkl} + Animal_{ijklm} + error_{ijklmn}$$

Heritability values greater than 0.3 indicate that the trait will have a high genetic effect trait for the offspring. Some performance heritability estimates in racing and equestrian sports are: 0.15 to 0.55 for flat gallop racing 0.20 to 0.40 for trot or pace racing, 0.18 to 0.19 for show jumping and three-day-eventing and 0.17 for dressage (Hintz, 1980). Note that heritability estimates are valid only for the breeds for which they were calculated and they should be recalculated periodically.

Muscle power: percentages of fast and slow Myosin Heavy Chains (MHC) of gluteus medius

MHC percentages were measured in small muscle samples of 20-30 mg collected by microbiopsy under local anesthesia. The analysis of slow MHC I and fast MHC IIA and IIX was performed using monoclonal antibodies with an ELISA method (Barrey *et al.*, 1999).

Muscular traits	Heritability	S.E.
Percentage of fast myosin heavy chain	I: 0.28; IIA & IIX: 0.13-0.28	0.1
Relative area of fibers	I: 0.23; IIA & IIX: 0.12- 0.15	0.1
Capillary density	0.20	0.09

Evaluation of cardiac and aerobic capacity

French trotters performed an exercise test at increasing speed. The heart rate and blood lactate were measured in order to determine the speed related changes of these variables. The speed eliciting 200 heart beats/min (V200) and a blood lactate concentration of 4 mmol/l (VLa4) were calculated.

Physiological traits	Heritability	S.E.
Cardiac capacity V200	0.46	0.11
Lactate anaerobic threshold VLa4	0.10	0.06

Gait analysis

To measure kinetic and temporal variables of the walk, trot, gallop and jump the horses were equipped with the gait analysis system Equimetrix ® (Barrey *et al.*, 1997; 2001; 2002). Two accelerometers were fixed with an elastic girth on the sternum. This ensured that the transducer was held close to the horse's centre of gravity. The device recorded the dorso-ventral, medio-lateral and longitudinal acceleration of the horse during the exercise and provided gait variables described in the following tables. Heritability estimates of canter, gallop and jumping variables, like take off impulse were rather high: 0.23 to 0.52 (Barrey *et al.*, 2002).

Gait variables	Walk h^2 (SE)	Trot h^2 (SE)	Canter h^2 (SE)
Stride characteristics			
Speed	0	0.30 (0.14)	NA
Stride length	0	0.29 (0.13)	NA
Stride frequency	0	0.20 (0.15)	0.32 (0.19)
Dorsoventral motion			
Symmetry	0.10 (0.08)	0.12 (0.08)	NA
Regularity	0.10 (0.13)	0.12 (0.09)	NA
Displacement	0.16 (0.12)	0.14 (0.08)	NA
Dorsoventral activity	0.41 (0.12)	0.22 (0.10)	0.50 (0.13)
Gait rhythm	0.29 (0.10)	0.05 (0.07)	NA
Longitudinal motion			
Mean propulsion vector	0.19 (0.07)	0.20 (0.11)	NA
Propulsion duration	0.69 (0.13)	0.38 (0.15)	NA
Longitudinal activity	0	0.44 (0.14)	0.46 (0.20)

h^2: Heritability; SE: standard error; NA: non available data.

Traits	Horse	Poney
Approach strides	0.34	0.41
Take off force	0.23	0.43
Jump flight	0.30	0.42
Landing force	0.52	0.40

Morphology

Using a two-dimensional image analysis system Equimetrix® it has been possible to measure French saddle horses and to calculate the heritability estimates of the main morphological traits. The conformation is poorly heritable in French saddle horses and more heritable in ponies. In both breeds these conformation traits are poorly related to the sport performances.

Traits	Horse	Poney
Height	0.16	0.56
Back	0.17-0.20	0.09-0.52
Hindlimb segments	0.15	0.31
Hindlimb angles	0.18	0.36
Forelimb segments	0.19	0.29
Forelimb angels	0.20	0.31

Conclusion

The gallop, trot and cardiac capacity variables have greater heritability estimates than VLa4 and muscular traits. However, the relationships with the performance should be taken into account. Muscular traits are significantly different between high and poor performers in racing and jumping horses. For harness trotters, the VLa4 is less heritable but more related to performance than V200. For equestrian sport horses, the use of gait variables like stride frequency, propulsion power and jump variables is better indicated for early selection. For racing horses muscular and cardiac capacity are the better parameters for early selection.

Take-off of the equine genomics with the recent horse genome publication

The equine genome has been sequenced and annotated by an international consortium (Wade *et al.*, 2009). The task has been conducted by the Broad Institute Sequencing Platform (Cambridge, MA, USA). All the database is available online at http://www.ncbi.nlm.nih.gov/genome/guide/horse/

This important information allows to produce new genetic investigations in various domains and to design new genomic tools such as single nucleotide polymorphism chips to detect gene markers or DNA microarrays to analyse the transcriptome expression and the regulation networks of genes. The summary of the original publication Genome Sequence, Comparative Analysis, and Population Genetics of the Domestic Horse is:

'We report a high-quality draft sequence of the genome of the horse (Equus caballus). The genome is relatively repetitive but has little segmental duplication. Chromosomes appear to have undergone few historical rearrangements: 53% of equine chromosomes show conserved synteny to a single human chromosome. Equine chromosome 11 is shown to have an evolutionary new centromere devoid of centromeric satellite DNA, suggesting that centromeric function may arise before satellite repeat accumulation. Linkage disequilibrium, showing the influences of early domestication of large herds of female horses, is intermediate in length between dog and human, and there is long-range haplotype sharing among breeds'.

Detecting the gene of performance and health factor using genotyping

Using the genome database, comparative genomics and genome-wide scan studies using SNP chips, it is now possible to identify some interesting genes linked to some performance traits like gallop distance ability or health troubles like osteochondrosis dissecans (OCD). Some small variations of the gene sequences like single nucleotide polymorphism SNP can be detected and the association to interesting trait can be demonstrated by statistical tests. This method has been applied in the two following studies.

Variants of the myostatin gene (MSTN) are associated with muscle hypertrophy phenotypes in a range of mammalian species, most notably cattle, dogs, mice, and humans. Using a sample of registered Thoroughbred horses, Hill *et al.* (2010) have identified a novel MSTN sequence polymorphism that is strongly associated with best race distance among elite racehorses. The authors observed that the SNP C/C horses are suited to fast, short-distance races; C/T horses compete favourably in middle-distance races; and T/T horses have greater stamina for longer distance. Evaluation of retrospective racecourse performance (n = 142) and stallion progeny performance predict that C/C and C/T horses are more likely to be successful two-year-old racehorses than T/T animals. This is the first SNP study which demonstrates a relationship between a racing performance trait and a specific gene variability.

Osteochondrosis dissecans is a major locomotor disorder in sport and racing horses. Several projects were started to detect genetic markers of this multifactorial joint disease affecting young horses. In a first study, Dierks *et al.* (2007) performed a genome-wide scan to detect quantitative trait loci (QTLs) for osteochondrosis (OC) and osteochondrosis dissecans (OCD) in horses. The genetic marker set comprised 260 microsatellites. Data were collected from 211 Hanoverian Warmblood horses consisting of 14 paternal half-sib families. Traits used were OC (fetlock and/or hock joints affected), OCD (fetlock and/or hock joints affected), fetlock OC, fetlock OCD, hock OC, and hock OCD. Genome-wide significant QTLs were located on equine chromosomes 2, 4, 5, and 16. QTLs for fetlock OC and hock OC partly overlapped on the same chromosomes, indicating that these traits may be genetically related. QTLs reached the chromosome-wide significance level on eight different equine chromosomes: 2, 3, 4, 5, 15, 16, 19 and 21. This whole-genome scan was a first step toward the identification of candidate genome regions harboring genes responsible for equine OC. In a second study, Lampe *et al.* (2009) used 29 microsatellite markers distributed in chromosome 5 to refine the map positions of the QTL already identified for OCD in the fetlock. Collagen type XXIV alpha 1 was identified as a potential functional candidate gene for equine osteochondrosis. This report is a further step towards unravelling the genes that cause equine fetlock osteochondrosis.

Using the new SNP Chip including 54602 markers (equine SNP50, Illumina®) distributed among the whole equine genome, other genome-wide scan projects are going on to detect SNP markers of show jumping and endurance race ability. Other projects are dealing with OCD and larynx paralysis in French saddle horses and Trotters.

Investigation of the phenotype by the analysis of gene expression and regulation

Gene expression and regulation determine most of the phenotype. The analysis of the cell transcriptome using DNA microarray provides qualitative and quantitative information about the up- and down-regulated pathways involved during exercise. The collected data are massive and complex and should be studied by sophisticated data mining methods in order to extract only the informative data. The first transcriptome studies in exercising horses were performed in the blood leucocytes of endurance horses (Barrey *et al.*, 2006) and in muscles of Thoroughbred racehorses in training (McGivney *et al.*, 2009). The following summaries explain the main results obtained.

1. Barrey *et al.* (2006) proposed to use cDNA microarrays in order to study the physiological adaptations and metabolic disorders in endurance horses. In order to show that genes are modulated in leucocytes in relationship with performance and clinical status of the horses, gene expression in leucocytes, haematological and biochemical parameters were compared between successful and disqualified endurance horses. Blood samples were collected at rest (TO) and just after a 140-160 km endurance race (T1) in 2 groups of

horses: 10 continuing successfully (S) and 10 disqualified horses stopped at a vet-gate for metabolic disorders (D). Total RNA was extracted from the blood cells (leucocytes), checked for purity, amplified and hybridised using mouse cDNA microarrays including 15,264 unique genes. Differential gene expressions were studied by hybridisation of each sample T1 vs. a control sample collected at TO (pool of 20 sound horses). Some significant differences were observed in the haematology and biochemistry of the 2 groups (S vs. D). In Group D, rhadomyolysis was confirmed with CK 13,124 u/l and AST 1,242 u/l. The list of 726 (including 603 annotated genes) significant genes was filtered according to a high P-value cut-off (P<0.00001). Among them, 130 were upregulated (expression ratio>1.5) and 288 were down-regulated (<1/1.5). Analysis of variance revealed 62 genes differentially expressed (P<0.05) in Groups D and S. The expression levels of 28 and 50 genes were significantly correlated (r>0.75) with CK and AST level in Group D, respectively. The gene ontology classification showed that more genes were up-regulated in S than in the D. More genes were down-regulated in the disqualified horses. Long exercise induced many significant gene modulations in leucocytes. Some genes were expressed in relationship with the clinical phenotype observed in Group D: rhabdomyolysis and haemolysis. Some of these genes could be candidates to explain poor performance or pathologies.

2. McGivney *et al.* (2009) suggested that exercise stimulates immediate early molecular responses as well as delayed responses during recovery, resulting in a return to homeostasis and enabling long-term adaptation. Global gene expression changes in equine skeletal muscle following exercise have not been reported. Therefore, to identify novel genes and key regulatory pathways responsible for exercise adaptation we have used equine-specific cDNA microarrays to examine global mRNA expression in skeletal muscle from a cohort of Thoroughbred horses (n=8) at three time points (before exercise, immediately post-exercise, and four hours post-exercise) following a single bout of treadmill exercise. Skeletal muscle biopsies were taken from the gluteus medius before (T0), immediately after (T1) and four hours after (T2) exercise. While only two genes had increased expression at T1 (P<0.05), by T2 932 genes had increased (P<0.05) and 562 genes had decreased expression (P<0.05). Functional analysis of genes differentially expressed during the recovery phase (T2) revealed an over-representation of genes localized to the actin cytoskeleton and with functions in the MAPK signalling, focal adhesion, insulin signalling, mTOR signaling, p53 signalling and Type II diabetes mellitus pathways. At T1, using a less stringent statistical approach it was observed an over-representation of genes involved in the stress response, metabolism and intracellular signalling. These findings suggest that protein synthesis, mechanosensation and muscle remodeling contribute to skeletal muscle adaptation towards improved integrity and hypertrophy. This is the

first study to characterize global mRNA expression profiles in equine skeletal muscle using an equine-specific microarray platform. Here novel genes and mechanisms are revealed that are temporally expressed following exercise providing new knowledge about the early and late molecular responses to exercise in the equine skeletal muscle transcriptome.

More recently, muscle diseases like the polysaccharide storage myopathy (PSSM) and recurrent exertional rhabdomyolysis (RER) were investigated using transcriptome analysis (Barrey *et al.*, 2009, 2010). Several cases of myopathies have been observed in the horse Norman Cob breed. Muscle histology examinations revealed that some families suffer from a polysaccharide storage myopathy (PSSM). It is assumed that a gene expression signature related to PSSM should be observed at the transcriptional level because the glycogen storage disease could also be linked to other dysfunctions in gene regulation. Thus, the functional genomic approach could be conducted in order to provide new knowledge about the metabolic disorders related to PSSM. It was proposed to explore the PSSM muscle fiber metabolic disorders by measuring gene expression in relationship with the histological phenotype. Genotypying analysis of GYS1 mutation revealed 2 homozygous (AA) and 5 heterozygous (GA) PSSM horses. In the PSSM muscles, histological data revealed PAS positive amylase resistant abnormal polysaccharides, inflammation, necrosis, and lipomatosis and active regeneration of fibers. Ultrastructural evaluation revealed a decrease of mitochondrial number and structural disorders. Extensive accumulation of an abnormal polysaccharide displaced and partially replaced mitochondria and myofibrils. The severity of the disease was higher in the two homozygous PSSM horses. Gene expression analysis revealed 129 genes significantly modulated ($P<0.05$). The following genes were up-regulated over 2 fold: IL18, CTSS, LUM, CD44, FN1, GST01. The most down-regulated genes were the following: mitochondrial tRNA, SLC2A2, PRKC alpha, VEGF alpha. Data mining analysis showed that protein synthesis, apoptosis, cellular movement, growth and proliferation were the main cellular functions significantly associated with the modulated genes ($P<0.05$). Several up-regulated genes, especially IL18, revealed a severe muscular inflammation in PSSM muscles. The up-regulation of glycogen synthase kinase-3 (GSK3beta) under its active form could be responsible for glycogen synthase (GYS1) inhibition and hypoxia-inducible factor (HIF1alpha) destabilization. The main disorders observed in PSSM muscles could be related to mitochondrial dysfunctions, glycogenesis inhibition and the chronic hypoxia of the PSSM muscles.

Conclusion: genomics perspective in equine exercise

With the great development of the genomic technologies many new applications will be soon available for the horse industry: candidate genes responsible of diseases and performance, genotyping, diagnostic tools and treatments. The first genotype test for racing distance ability is now available for flat racing. The diagnostic of PSSM myopathy by genotyping is routinely applied. Within five years, other genotyping methods will be available for early performance evaluation. Maybe new genomic treatment will be designed to treat some myopathies or other metabolic diseases as it is now applied in humans. The drawback of the biotech availability will be illicit use for doping using muscular transgenesis for example. Hopefully, research projects are already going on to detect this new type of genomic doping both in humans and animals.

References

Barrey, E. *et al.* (2010) Muscular microRNA expressions in healty and myopathic horses suffering from polysaccharide storage myopathy or recurrent exercise rhabdomyolysis. Abstract Booklet of the 8th International Conference on Equine Exercise Physiology, November 2010, Cape Town, South Africa.

Barrey, E., Desliens, F., Poirel, D., Biau, S., Lemaire, S., Rivero, J.L., Langlois, B. (2002). Early evaluation of dressage ability in different breeds. Eq Vet J Suppl 34, 319-324.

Barrey, E., Evans, S.E., Evans, D.L., Curtis, R.A., Quinton, R., Rose, R.J. (2001). Locomotion evaluation for racing in thoroughbreds. Eq Vet J Suppl 33, 99-103.

Barrey, E., Galloux, P. (1997). Analysis of the equine jumping technique by accelerometry. Eq Vet J Suppl 23, 45-49.

Barrey, E., Mucher, E., Jeansoule, N., Larcher, T., Guigand, L., Herszberg, B., Chaffaux, S., Guérin, G., Mata, X., Benech, P., Canale, M., Alibert, O., Maltere, P., Gidrol, X. (2009). Gene expression profiling in equine polysaccharide storage myopathy revealed inflammation, glycogenesis inhibition, hypoxia and mitochondrial dysfunctions. BMC Vet Res Aug 7, 5, 29.

Barrey, E., Mucher, E., Robert, C., Amiot, F., Gidrol, X. (2006). Gene expression profiling in blood cells of endurance horses completing competition or disqualified due to metabolic disorder. Eq Vet J Suppl 36, 43-49.

Barrey, E., Valette, J.P., Jouglin, M., Blouin, C., Langlois, B. (1999). Heritability of percentage of fast myosin heavy chains in skeletal muscles and relationship with performance. Eq Vet J Suppl 30, 289-292.

Barrey, E., Desliens, F., Blouin, C., Langlois, B. (2002). Proc of '28ème Journée d'étude', Les Haras nationaux, 27 Février, pp 157-176.

Dierks, C., Löhring, K., Lampe, V., Wittwer, C., Drögemüller, C., Distl, O. (2007). Genome-wide search for markers associated with osteochondrosis in Hanoverian warmblood horses. Mamm Genome 18, 739-747.

Hill, E.W., Gu, J., Eivers, S.S., Fonseca, R.G., McGivney, B.A., Govindarajan, P., Orr, N., Katz, L.M., MacHugh, D.A. (2010). Sequence polymorphism in MSTN predicts sprinting ability and racing stamina in thoroughbred horses. PLoS One Jan 20, 5 (1), e8645.

Hintz, R.L. (1980). Genetics of Performance in the Horse. J Anim Sci 51, 582-594.

Lampe, V., Dierks, C., Distl, O. (2009). Refinement of a quantitative trait locus on equine chromosome 5 responsible for fetlock osteochondrosis in Hanoverian warmblood horses. Anim Genet Aug 40, 553-555.

McGivney, B.A., Eivers, S.S., MacHugh, D.E., MacLeod, J.N., O'Gorman, G.M., Park, S.D., Katz, L.M., Hill, E.W. (2009). Transcriptional adaptations following exercise in thoroughbred horse skeletal muscle highlights molecular mechanisms that lead to muscle hypertrophy. BMC Genomics Dec 30,10, 638.

Wade, C.M., Giulotto, E., Sigurdsson, S., Zoli, M., Gnerre, S., Imsland, F., Lear, T.L., Adelson, D.L., Bailey, E., Bellone, R.R., Blöcker, H., Distl, O., Edgar, R.C., Garber, M., Leeb, T., Mauceli, E., MacLeod, J.N., Penedo, M.C., Raison, J.M., Sharpe, T., Vogel, J., Andersson, L., Antczak, D.F., Biagi, T., Binns, M.M., Chowdhary, B.P., Coleman, S.J., Della Valle, G., Fryc, S., Guérin, G., Hasegawa, T., Hill, E.W., Jurka, J., Kiialainen, A., Lindgren, G., Liu, J., Magnani, E., Mickelson, J.R., Murray, J., Nergadze, S.G., Onofrio, R., Pedroni, S., Piras, M.F., Raudsepp, T., Rocchi, M., Røed, K.H., Ryder, O.A., Searle, S., Skow, L., Swinburne, J.E., Syvänen, A.C., Tozaki, T., Valberg, S.J., Vaudin, M., White, J.R., Zody, M.C.; Broad Institute Genome Sequencing Platform; Broad Institute Whole Genome Assembly Team, Lander, E.S., Lindblad-Toh, K. (2009). Genome sequence, comparative analysis, and population genetics of the domestic horse. Science 326 (5954), 865-867.

Equine osteochondrosis: what can genetics tell the breeder and rider

Ottmar Distl
Institute of Animal Breeding and Genetics, University of Veterinary Medicine Hannover, Bünteweg 17p, 30559 Hannover, Germany

Abstract

Osteochondrosis (OC) is a developmental disease in growing individuals due to disturbed differentiation and maturation of cartilage particularly at predilection sites of the fetlock, hock and stifle joints. Recent studies have shown high prevalences of OC in the limb joints of young riding horses. Horses with radiographically visible osteochondrotic lesions are at a higher risk of developing orthopaedic problems later in life than unaffected horses. This paper provides a brief overview of prevalences and heritabilities for OC and perspectives for selection in the horse industry. We describe molecular genetic approaches to equine osteochondrosis. Whole genome scans and genome-wide association analyses for quantitative trait loci (QTL) and comparative genomics using candidate genes may lead to new insights into the molecular mechanisms of pathogenesis of osteochondrosis and to gene tests for OC in horses.

Introduction

Osteochondrosis (OC) is caused by a disturbance of the endochondral ossification of growing cartilage of the articular/epiphyseal complex (Jeffcott, 1996; Rooney, 1979; Van De Lest *et al.*, 1999). Cartilage cells appear to proliferate normally, but maturation and differentiation are abnormal in OC (Trotter and McIlwraith, 1981). The loss of normal differentiation of cartilage cells means that transitional calcification of the matrix does not occur and that capillary sprouts can not penetrate the distal region of the hypertrophic zone (Dämmrich, 1985; Shingleton *et al.*, 1997). The altered process of endochondral ossification leads to retention and thickening of cartilage, resulting in the development of a cartilage core. These primary lesions can progress to further damage within the joint so that signs, such as subchondral fractures, subchondral cyst-like lesions, cartilage flaps, separation of osteochondral fragments (joint mice, chips, corpora libera, osteochondritis dissecans, OCD), osteochondritis and synovitis, can occur (Dämmrich, 1985; Jeffcott, 1991; Nixon, 1990). Articulations of the limbs mainly affected by this developmental disease are the fetlock, hock, and stifle joints (Jeffcott, 1991). Radiographic signs consistent with OC are irregular texture of the bone with variable radiopacity (e.g. radioluceny of the subchondral bone) and changes of the regular bone contour such as smoothly flattened, irregularly flattened and smaller or larger concavity or isolated radiodense areas at specific sites of the predisposed joints. The predilection sites in hock joints are the intermediate ridge of the distal tibia, the lateral/medial trochlear ridge of the talus and the lateral/medial malleolus of the tibia (Trotter and McIlwraith, 1981; Kroll *et al.*, 2001). In the stifle joints, the predilection sites are the lateral/medial trochlear ridge of the femur, the trochlear groove of the femur and the patella. The predilection site in the fetlock joint for OC is the dorsal aspect of the sagittal ridge of the 3rd metacarpal/metatarsal bone. There is no common opinion whether the dorsoproximal rim of the proximal phalanx should be classified as predilection site for OC in horses. In trotters, and coldblood horses palmar/plantar fragments and/or bone defects at the site of attachment of the short sesamoidean ligaments to the proximal phalanx (POFs) are often seen (Carlsten *et al.*, 1993; Grøndahl and Dolvik, 1993) and these changes were genetically correlated with OC in coldblood horses (Wittwer *et al.*, 2007a). The intervertebral articular processes of the cervical spine are most commonly affected in the vertebral joints (Van Weeren and Barnefeld, 1999).

OC occurs in many different livestock species and belongs to those diseases of the locomotory system frequently detected radiographically in young horses (Arnan and Hertsch, 2005; Carlsten *et al.*, 1993; Hoppe, 1984; Wittwer *et al.*, 2006). The specific causes are still unknown but OC appears to be multifactorial in origin (Jeffcott, 1991; Van Weeren, 2005).

The present paper gives an overview of the prevalences and heritabilities of OC in fetlock and hock joints of different horse breeds. The recently identified quantitative trait loci (QTL) for equine OC will be discussed in respect to positional candidate genes and in addition, the release of the horse genome assembly new developments genomics useful for identifying responsible genes for OC will be presented.

Prevalence of OC

Reports on the prevalence indicate that OC is present in warmblood and trotter horse populations at frequencies between 10 and 64% across a range of different breeds (Jeffcott, 1991; Philipsson *et al.*, 1993; Stock *et al.*, 2005a, 2005b; Willms *et al.*, 1999; Winter *et al.*, 1996) (Table 1). The large differences may be attributed to the different definitions of the osteochondrotic findings. Osteochondrotic lesions have been often referred to traumatic origin or to the osteochondrosis syndrome, in dependence of the location of the radiographic signs (Jeffcott and Henson, 1998; Jeffcott, 1991). In the case of radiographic findings at the dorsoproximal aspect of the third phalanx or in the palmar/plantar region of the fetlock joint it is more difficult to distinguish between presumably traumatic and osteochondrotic origin. Grøndahl and Dolvik (1993)

Table 1. Prevalence of osteochondrosis and osteochondral fragments in limb joints of horses by breed and age.

Horse population/age	Affected joint / osteochondral findings	Affected	References
Danish trotters (n=325), 18 months to 2 years	Hock: Osteochondral fragments at intermediate ridge of distal tibia	12.0%	Schougaard *et al.*, 1990
Draft horses (n=51), 1-43 months	Fetlock: Fragmentation of the sagittal ridge of McIII[1] Hock: Osteochondritis dissecans of the distal intermediate ridge Hock: Osteochondritis dissecans of the lateral trochlear ridge of the talus	1.0% 10.2% 7.1%	Riley *et al.*, 1998
Dutch Warmblood horses (n=590), 3 years	Hock: No specification	13.7%	KWPN, 1994
Swedish Standardbred trotters (foals, n=77), 1-16 months	Fetlock: POF[2] and UPE[3] Fetlock: DF[d] Fetlock: Abnormal enchondral ossification Hock: Bony fragment with or without defect in underlying bone or subchondral bone defect >5mm	14.3% 2.6% 24.7% 10.4%	Carlsten *et al.*, 1993
Swedish Standardbred trotters (n=674), 11-24 months	Fetlock: POF[2] Fetlock: UPE[3] Fetlock: DF[4] Hock: Bony fragment with or without defect in underlying bone or subchondral bone defect >5 mm	21.5% 4.2% 4.4% 10.5%	Philipsson *et al.*, 1993
Italian Maremmano horses (n=350), 2-3 years	Fetlock: OF[5] Fetlock: OF[5] at sagittal ridge of McIII[a] Fetlock: OF[5] at dorsal margin of foreleg proximal phalanx Hock: OF[5] Hock: OF[5] at distal intermediate ridge of tibia Hock: OF[5] at medial malleolus Hock: OF[5] at lateral malleolus	2.8% 0.8% 2.0% 9.2% 8.3% 0.3% 0.6%	Pieramati *et al.*, 2003
Norwegian trotters (n=753), 6-21 months	Fetlock: POF[2] Fetlock: UPE[3] Fetlock: DF[4] Hock: OCD in tibiotarsal joints Hock: Bony fragment with or without defect in underlying bone or subchondral bone defect >5 mm Hock: DBT Hock: Defect(s) at lateral trochlea talus	11.8% 2.4% 4.8% 14.3% 12.5% 1.7% 1.1%	Grøndahl and Dolvik, 1993

Table 1. Continued.

Horse population/age	Affected joint / osteochondral findings	Affected	References
Holstein horses (mares, n=456), 6 months to 2 years	Hock: OCD tarsi (no specification)	34 - 64%	Willms *et al.*, 1999
Holstein horses (foals, n=144), 6 months	Hock: OCD tarsi (no specification)	19 - 58%	Willms *et al.*, 1999
German Warmblood (suckling foals, n=130)	Fetlock: Osseous fragments at the dorsal aspect of the 3rd metacarpal/metatarsal bone Fetlock: Palmar/plantar osseous fragments of the proximal phalanx Fetlock: Osteochondrotic findings at the dorsal aspect of the 3rd metacarpal/metatarsal bone Hock: Osseous fragments in talocrural joints Hock: Osteochondrotic findings in talocrural joints	14.6% 17.7% 37.7% 10.7% 82.3%	Kroll *et al.*, 2001
German Warmblood horses (n=3566), 3-8 years	Fetlock, Hock: Osteochondrosis dissecans (no specification)	11.0%	Winter *et al.*, 1996
Hanoverian Warmblood horses (n=3749), 3-7 years	Fetlock: Isolated radiopaque area Fetlock, front limbs: Isolated radiopaque area Fetlock, hind limbs: Isolated radiopaque area Hock: Isolated radiopaque area in talocrural joints	20.7% 9.5% 13.7% 9.6%	Stock *et al.*, 2005a, b
South German Coldblood horses (n=167)	Fetlock: Osteochondrotic findings at the dorsal aspect of the 3rd metacarpal/metatarsal bone Fetlock: Osseous fragments at the dorsal aspect of the 3rd metacarpal/metatarsal bone Fetlock: Palmar/plantar osseous fragments Hock: Osteochondrotic findings in talocrural joints	53.9% 26.4% 16.2% 40.1%	Wittwer *et al.*, 2007a

[1] Third metacarpal/metatarsal bone.
[2] Palmar/plantar osseous fragment and/or bone defect >5 mm at attachment site of short sesmoidean ligament.
[3] Ununited palmar/plantar eminence of proximal phalanx (including intra- and extra-articular fragments).
[4] Dorsal fragment(s) at dorsoproximal rim of proximal phalanx and/or fragments(s) or defects >5 mm at dorsal part of sagittal ridge of distal third metacarpal/metatarsal bone.
[5] Osteochondral fragment.

distinguished between OC in hock joints as bony fragments at the intermediate ridge of the distal tibia and/or at the trochlea of the talus and POFs in fetlock joints at the attachment site of the short sesamoidean ligaments, excluding bony fragments at the dorsoproximal end of the proximal phalanx. Schougaard *et al.* (1990) investigated osteochondral fragments with or without defects at different locations in hock joints, excluding defects without osteochondral fragments. Pieramati *et al.* (2003) regarded osteochondral fragments at different locations of fetlock and hock joints. Kroll *et al.* (2001) distinguished between osteochondral lesions, such as isolated radiopaque areas, irregularities and low density of bone margins at the dorsal aspect of the sagittal ridge of the 3rd metacarpal/metatarsal bone, and in the distal part of the tibia and the lateral trochlea tali.

In South German Coldblood horses the prevalence of OC was sharply increasing at an age of about twelve months. The most frequently affected animals were at an age of between 10 and 17 months and half of the foals that were x-rayed twice, showed signs of OC only in the second examination at an age of about 25 months (Wittwer *et al.*, 2006).

Heritability of OC

It is generally accepted that genetic components play a large role in the etiology of the OC syndrome (Grøndahl and Dolvik, 1993; Jeffcott, 1991; Philipsson *et al.*, 1993; Pieramati *et al.*, 2003; Stock *et al.*, 2005b; Willms *et al.*, 1999; Winter *et al.*, 1996). The relative importance of additive genetic variation is determined by the heritability in the narrow sense which quantifies the degree to which phenotypic variance is explained by additive genetic variance. Heritability estimates are population-specific parameters and in addition, depend on the type of method used and on the familial structure and group of relatives used for estimation. Sire models do not account for relationships other than paternal half-sibs and do not use all information available. The animal model overcomes these shortcomings and thus, is now most commonly employed in animal breeding. Animal models use information on all relatives of an animal without reduction to specific structures of relatives. In the case of categorical data, a threshold model or a transformation onto the underlying distribution has to be applied in order to avoid underestimation of heritabilities. The heritability estimates for OC in Warmblood horses were between 0.10 and 0.34 when threshold models were applied and the additive genetic effect of the animal was included in the model (Table 2). In some cases the estimates have high standard errors due to low numbers of animals with phenotypic records and these estimates are not significantly different from zero (KWPN, 1994; Pieramati *et al.*, 2003). The heritability estimates in studies in trotters vary between 0.17 and 0.52 (Grøndahl and Dolvik, 1993; Philipsson *et al.*, 1993; Schougaard *et al.*, 1990). The reasons for these large differences may be because of the type of method

Table 2. Heritability estimates for equine osteochondrosis in different limb joints by horse breeds.

Population and number of investigated horses	Radiographic finding	Heritability estimate	Method of analysis	References
Danish trotters (n=325)	OF[1] (hock)	0.26 ± 0.14	STM[6]	Schougaard *et al.*, 1987
Norwegian trotters (n=644)	POF[3] (fetlock) OC[2] (hock)	0.52 0.21	STM[6] (REML[7])	Grøndahl and Dolvik,1993
Swedish trotters (n=793)	OC[2] (hock) POF[3] (fetlock)	0.27 0.24	LSM[8] (DL[9])	Philipsson *et al.*, 1993
Maremmano horses (n=350)	DOF[4] (fetlock) OF[1] (hock)	0.13-0.14 ± 0.22-0.23	LAM[10] (REML[7], DL[9])	Pieramati *et al.*, 2003
Dutch warmblood (mares; n=590)	OF[1] (hock)	0.14 ± 0.17	LAM[10] (REML[7], DL[9])	KWPN, 1994
Hanoverian warmblood (n=3725)	OF[1] (fetlock) OF[1] (hock)	0.19 ± 0.03 0.37 ± 0.06	LAM[10] (REML[7], DL[9])	Stock *et al.*, 2005b
German riding horses (n=2407)	OCD[5] (hock)	0.07 ± 0.03	LAM[10] (REML[7])	Winter *et al.*, 1996
Holsteiner horses (mares; n=456)	OCD[5] (hock)	0.34 ± 0.06	ATM[11] (GS[12])	Willms *et al.*, 1999
Holsteiner horses (foals; n=144)	OCD[5] (hock)	0.19 ± 0.02	ATM[11] (GS[12])	Willms *et al.*, 1999
Hanoverian WB (n=624)	OC (hock) OC (fetlock) OCD (hock) OCD (fetlock)	0.08±0.05 0.07±0.08 0.10±0.05 0.15±0.07	LAM[10] (REML[7])	Schober, 2003
Dutch WB (n=811)	OC (stifle) OC (hock) OC (fetlock) OCD (stifle) OCD (hock) OCD (fetlock)	0.07±0.06 0.15±0.08 0.08±0.10 0.02±0.04 0.26±0.09 0.06±0.07	LAM[10] (REML[7])	Van Grevenhof *et al.*, 2009
South German Coldblood (n=167)	OC (hock) OC (fetlock) OCD (fetlock)	0.04±0.07 0.16±0.16 0.08±0.09	LAM[10] (REML[7], DL[9])	Wittwer *et al.*, 2007a

[1] Osteochondral fragments. [2] Osteochondrosis. [3] Palmar/plantar osteochondral fragments. [4] Dorsal osteochondral fragmentation. [5] Osteochondrosis dissecans. [6] Sire threshold model. [7] Residual Maximum Likelihood. [8] Linear sire model. [9] Dempster Lerner transformation onto the liability model. [10] Linear animal model. [11] Animal threshold model. [12] Gibbs sampling.

applied for estimation (sire model instead of an animal model), the horse breed investigated, differing data structures, and in some studies, the low numbers of animals included. Using a sire threshold model, a heritability of 0.26 was estimated, based on 325 yearlings representing the majority of the progeny of nine trotter stallions (Schougaard *et al.*, 1990). In Swedish trotters a heritability of h^2=0.27 was estimated for radiographic findings of OC in hock joints with 793 horses under examination (Philipsson *et al.*, 1993). Heritability estimates of 0.21 for hock joints were estimated for 644 trotters that were progeny from 39 sires (Grøndahl and Dolvik, 1993).

In several reports the considered locations of OC lesions in the joints were not specified and there were different definitions of osteochondrosis for the examined locations. Heritability estimations were mostly confined to hock OC (Carlsten *et al.*, 1993; Grøndahl and Dolvik, 1993; KWPN, 1994; Philipsson *et al.*, 1993; Schougaard *et al.*, 1987; Willms *et al.*, 1999; Winter *et al.*, 1996) or to osteochondral fragments in hock and fetlock joints (Stock *et al.*, 2005b). Partly, no specification was made which joints are taken in consideration (KWPN, 1994; Willms *et al.*, 1999; Winter *et al.*, 1996). Genetic analyses using radiographs from 624 foals at an age between four and nine months and radiographs from the same could demonstrate genetic correlations among signs for osteochondrotic lesions in foals and OCD (joint bodies at the predilection sites in horses aged two years) at r_g=0.84 for fetlock joints and r_g=0.99 for hock joints (Schober, 2003). The corresponding phenotypic correlations were r_p=0.66 (fetlock joints) and r_p=0.68 (hock joints) indicating a significant consistency of the radiological findings for the two different age classes. The genetic correlations between osseous fragments in fetlock and hock joints were slightly to moderately negative in warmblood horses (Stock *et al.*, 2005b).

The heritabilities reported indicate that the selection response is high enough to employ selection programmes based on breeding values for OC. Currently breeding values are predicted for performance traits in animal models for several warmblood populations in Europe. Accordingly, radiographic data recorded for a larger number of horses have to be provided for the genetic evaluation of OC in sires and dams. The radiographic examination of the equine limbs has become a common feature at riding horse auctions and at stallion performance tests, but needs further implementation in performance tests for mares. This way a sufficient amount of data could be collected to predict breeding values for OC with sufficient reliability. Presuming the availability of sufficient data, breeding values can already be predicted for young horses presented for studbook inspection or stallion licensing. Therefore, parameters of the health of the equine skeleton could be considered at this early stage of selection of breeding animals. A study including radiographs of 5,928 Hanoverian warmblood horses and their relationship matrix containing 23,662 horses from four generations could show the feasibility of selection schemes that simultaneously accounted for performance traits and for the most prevalent radiographic findings influencing the health of the equine skeleton (Stock and Distl, 2005). Conditions for limb health regarded were osseous fragments in fetlock and hock joints, deforming arthropathy in hock joints and pathologic changes in navicular bones. Breeding values were predicted for these radiographic findings and then selection indices developed which included the aforementioned radiographic traits, dressage and jumping traits with different weights. When weighing radiographic traits with 30-60% as opposed to the respective performance traits, and selecting only sires with above-average total indices, the prevalence of each radiographic finding considered was lowered by up to 10% in the progeny. Considering only one radiographic finding at a time, the maximum attainable response to selection in a generation was a decrease of prevalences of radiographic findings by 31-52% (Stock and Distl, 2005).

Quantitative trait loci for OC

In recent years, there have been major advances in mapping the equine genome. A whole-genome radiation hybrid map (Chowdhary *et al.*, 2003), comprehensive genetic linkage maps (Swinburne *et al.*, 2000, 2006), a medium-density horse gene map (Perrocheau *et al.*, 2006) and informative marker sets (Mittman *et al.*, 2010) have been developed.

Equine maps with a large number of highly polymorphic markers equidistantly distributed over the whole genome are prerequisites to perform linkage studies for identifying quantitative trait loci (QTL). QTL are genomic regions which are highly likely to harbour genes influencing the trait of interest. The larger the proportion of the phenotypic variation of a polygenic or multifactorial trait the more useful the QTL are for selection. QTL show linkage disequilibrium within families or in the whole population. An ideal marker for a QTL shows linkage disequilibrium in the whole population. After identification of QTL in population-wide linkage disequilibrium marker assisted selection provides the possibility to improve accuracy of selection in young horses and to shorten the generation interval in horse breeding.

Whole-genome scans for half-sib families with a high incidence of OC were employed to detect QTL significantly contributing to the phenotypic expression of OC. Data from 14 half-sib families of Hanoverian Warmblood horses were analysed using microsatellite markers to detect quantitative trait loci (QTL) with significant influence on the development of OC (Dierks *et al.*, 2007) genome-wide significant. QTL for osteochondrosis in fetlock and hock joints were found on horse chromosomes (ECA) 2, 4, 5, and 16. Further chromosome-wide significant QTL were located on horse chromosomes 3, 15, 19 and 21. QTL for fetlock OC were on ECA 2, 4 and 5. The locations of QTL for hock OC were on ECA2, 15, 16 and 21. In a population of South German coldblood horses a whole genome scan for OC was carried out (Wittwer *et al.*, 2007b). In total, 10 chromosome-wide significant QTL were found on different equine chromosomes with influence on the development of OC in fetlock and hock joints. Using the human-equine comparative maps (Chowdhary *et al.* 2003, Perrocheau *et al.* 2006) the positions of the QTL for OC can be compared with QTL or locations of genes implicated in osteoarthritis or growth in humans.

In order to refine those identified QTL, an extended marker set containing published as well as newly developed microsatellites and SNPs was used. Fine mapping confirmed QTL on ECA2, 4, 5, 16, and 21 (Lampe *et al.* 2009b, 2009c; unpublished results). On ECA18, a new QTL could be identified in Hanoverian warmblood horses (Lampe *et al.* 2009a). On ECA2, a SNP within the *neurochondrin* (*NCDN*) gene was significantly associated with OC traits. On ECA4, three significantly associated SNPs have been identified within the genome-wide significant OC-QTL region, whereof two SNPs were located in intergenic regions and one SNP was in intron 2 of the *HECT, C2 and WW domain containing E3 ubiquitin protein ligase 1* (*HECW1*) gene.

In South German Coldblood horses, a whole genome scan was performed for the same traits as for Hanoverian warmblood horses and additionally for palmar/plantar osseous fragments (POFs). Heritability of POFs implicated a genetic component in the variation of the development of osteochondrosis (Wittwer *et al.* 2007a). The genome scan included 250 polymorphic microsatellites equally distributed over all chromosomes with a mean distance of 17.7 cM with an enhanced use of microsatellites in putative QTL regions. Chromosome-wide significant QTL were found on 10 chromosomes, including seven QTL for fetlock OC and one QTL on ECA18 for hock OC and fetlock OC. Significant QTL for POFs in fetlock joints were located on equine chromosomes 1, 4, 8, 12 and 18. On ECA4, the QTL for POFs reached the genome-wide significance level (Wittwer *et al.* 2007b). On ECA4, significantly associated SNPs in the *acyloxyacyl hydrolase* (*AOAH*) gene could be identified (Wittwer *et al.* 2008). On ECA18, Wittwer *et al.* (2009) found a significantly associated intronic SNP in the *xin actin-binding repeat containing 2* (*XIRP2*) gene.

Since 2008, a commercially available SNP microarray containing more than 50,000 SNPs enables genome-wide association analyses, quantitative trait loci (QTL) identification and additionally QTL validation. The equine SNP50 Genotyping BeadChip was developed by Illumina in collaboration with the International Equine Genome Mapping Workshop and the Morris Animal Foundation's Equine Genome Consortium. Researchers around the globe use the equine SNP chip to investigate common single gene defects and multigenic diseases including musculoskeletal, neuromuscular, cardiovascular and respiratory disorders. In order to prove detected QTL of OC in Hanoverian warmblood horses, a genome-wide association analysis (GWA) was performed using about 300 Hanoverian horses. This GWA study confirmed the previously known QTL on horse chromosomes and furthermore, new QTL on ECA3, 7, 19, 20, 22, 26 and 29 could be detected. Consequently, these associated SNPs can be used for developing genomic breeding values for Hanoverian horses. The microarray technology opens great improvements towards unravelling genes underlying QTL for equine OC and therefore, the development of genome-wide tests for OC.

Conclusions

Osteochondrosis is one of the most common joint diseases in growing horses. The aetiology of OC in the horse is still not fully understood, but more research has focused on the molecular mechanisms involved. The substantial progress of comparative genomics, the recently initiated horse genome project in Lower-Saxony (Distl and Blöcker, 2005; http://www.volkswagenstiftung.de/presse-news/presse05/108122005.pdf) and the horse whole genome sequencing project of the Broad Institute at MIT (Wade *et al.*, 2009) provide a very effective approach towards unravelling the genetic basis of equine OC. The genomic regions of QTL for OC identified by whole genome scans and genome-wide association analyses can now be used for fine mapping using horse genome sequences and comparative genomics. Due to these new developments in horse genomics and application of next-generation-sequencing for fine-mapping, the further refinement of the QTL positions identified and unravelling of genes responsible for OC will be progress very fast.

References

Arnan, P., Hertsch, B. (2005). OCD des Fessel-, Sprung- und Kniegelenks im Vergleich vom Fohlen zum Zweijährigen. Pferdeheilkunde 21, 322-326.

Dierks, C., Löhring, K., Wittwer, C., Drögemüller, C., Distl, O. (2006). Genome-wide search for markers associated with osteochondrosis in Hanoverian warmblood horses. Mammalian Genome 18, 739-747.

Carlsten, J., Sandgren, B., Dalin, G. (1993). Development of osteochondrosis in the tarsocrural joint and osteochondral fragments in the fetlock joints of Standardbred trotters. I. A radiological survey. Equine veterinary Journal Supplement 16, 42-47.

Chowdhary, B.P., Raudsepp, T., Kata, S.R., Goh, G., Millon, L.V., Allan, V., PiumI, F., Guerin, G., Swinburne, J., Binns, M., Lear, T.L., Mickelson, J., Murray, J., Antczak, D.F., Womack, J.E., Skow, L.C. (2003). The first-generation whole-genome radiation hybrid map in the horse identifies conserved segments in human and mouse genomes. Genome Research 13, 742-751.

Dämmrich, K. (1985). Wachstumsstörungen des Skeletts bei jungen Pferden. Pferdeheilkunde 1, 5-13.

Distl, O., Blöcker, H. (2005). http://www.volkswagenstiftung.de/presse-news/presse05/108122005.pdf.

Grøndahl, A.M., Dolvik, N.I. (1993). Heritability estimations of osteochondrosis in the tibiotarsal joint and of bony fragments in the palmar/plantar portion of the metacarpo- and metatarsophalangeal joints of horses. Journal of the American Veterinary Medical Association 203, 101-104.

Hoppe, F. (1984). Radiological investigations of osteochondrosis dissecans in Standardbred trotters and Swedish Warmblood horses. Equine veterinary Journal Supplement 16, 425-429.

Jeffcott, L.B. (1991). Osteochondrosis in the horse-searching for the key to pathogenesis. Equine veterinary Journal 23, 331-338.

Jeffcott, L.B. (1996). Osteochondrosis – an international problem for the horse industry. Journal of Equine Veterinary Science 16, 32-37.

Jeffcott, L.B., Henson, F.M.D. (1998). Studies on growth cartilage in the horse and their application to aetiopathogenesis of dyschondroplasia (osteochondrosis). The Veterinary Journal 156, 177-192.

Kroll, A., Hertsch, B., Höppner, S. (2001). Entwicklung osteochondraler Veränderungen in Fessel- und Talokruralgelenken im Röntgenbild beim Fohlen. Pferdeheilkunde 17, 489-500.

KWPN (1994). The frequency and heredity of navicular disease, sesamoidosis, fetlock joint arthrosis, bone spavin, osteochondrosis of the hock. A radiographic progeny study. KWPN (Koninklijke Vereniging Warmbloed Paardenstamboek Nederland), Zeist.

Lampe, V., Dierks, C., Komm, K., Distl, O. (2009a). Identification of a new quantitative trait locus on equine chromosome 18 responsible for osteochondrosis in Hanoverian warmblood horses. Journal of Animal Science 87, 3477-3481.

Lampe, V., Dierks, C., Distl, O. (2009b). Refinement of a quantitative trait locus on equine chromosome 5 responsible for fetlock osteochondrosis in Hanoverian warmblood horses. Animal Genetics 40, 553-555.

Lampe, V., Dierks, C., Distl, O. (2009c). Refinement of a quantitative gene locus on equine chromosome 16 responsible for osteochondrosis in Hanoverian warmblood horses. Animal 3, 1224-1231.

Mittmann, E.H., Lampe, V., Mömke, S., Zeitz, A., Distl, O. (2010). Characterization of a minimal microsatellite set for whole genome scans informative in warmblood and coldblood horse breeds. Journal of Heredity 101, 246-250.

Nixon, A.J. (1990). Osteochondrosis and osteochondritis dissecans of the equine fetlock. Compendium Continuing Education Practice Veterinary 12, 1463-1475.

Perrocheau, M., Boutreux, V., Chadi, S., Mata, X., Decaunes, P., Raudsepp, T., Durkin, K., Incarnato, D., Iannuzzi, L., Lear, T.L., Hirota, K., Hasegawa, T., Zhu, B., de Jong, P., Cribiu, E.P., Chowdhary, B.P., Guérin, G. (2006). Construction of a medium-density horse gene map. Animal Genetics 37, 145-155.

Philipsson, J., Andreasson, E., Sandgren, B., Dalin, G., Carlsten, J. (1993). Osteochondrosis in the tarsocrural joint and osteochondral fragments in the fetlock joints in Standardbred trotters. II. Heritybility. Equine veterinary Journal Supplement 16, 38-41.

Pieramati, C., Pepe, M., Silvestrelli, M., Bolla, A. (2003). Heritability estimation of osteochondrosis dissecans in Maremmano horses. Livestock Production Science 79, 249-255.

Riley, C.B., Scott, W.M., Caron, J.P., Fretz, P.B., Bailey, J.V., Barber, S.M. (1998). Osteochondritis dessicans and subchondral cystic lesions in draft horses: A retrospective study. Canadian Veterinary Journal 39, 627-633.

Rooney, J.R. (1979). Osteochondrosis in the horse. Modern Veterinary Practice 56, 41-43.

Schober, M. (2003). Schätzung von genetischen Effekten beim Auftreten von Osteochondrosis dissecans beim Warmblutpferd. Dissertation, Georg-August-Universität-Göttingen.

Schougaard, H., Ronne, J.F., Philipsson, J. (1987). Incidence and inheritance of osteochondrosis in the sport horse. 38th Annual Meeting EAAP, 28 September to 1 October 1987, Lisboa, Portugal.

Schougaard, H., Ronne, J.F., Philipsson, J. (1990). A radiographic survey of tibiotarsal osteochondrosis in a selected population of trotting horses in Denmark and its possible genetic significance. Equine veterinary Journal 22, 288-289.

Shingleton, W.D., Mackie, E.W., Cawston, T.E., Jeffcott, L.B. (1997). Cartilage canals in equine articular/epiphyseal growth cartilage and a possible association with dyschondroplasia. Equine veterinary Journal 29, 360-364.

Stock, K.F., Distl, O. (2005). Prediction of breeding values for osseus fragments in fetlock and hock joints, deforming arthropathy in hock joints and pathologic changes in the nacivular bones of Hanoverian Warmblood horses. Livest. Prod. Sci. 92, 77-94.

Stock K.F., Hamann H., Distl O. (2005a). Prevalence of osseous fragments in limb joints of Hanoverian Warmblood horses. Journal of Veterinary Medicine A 52, 388-394.

Stock K.F., Hamann H., Distl O. (2005b). Estimation of genetic parameters for the prevalence of osseous fragments in limb joints of Hanoverian Warmblood horses. Journal of Animal Breeding and Genetics 122, 271-280.

Swinburne, J.E., Gerstenberg, C., Breen, M., Aldridge, V., Lockhart, L., Marti, E., Antczak, D., Eggleston-Stott, M., Bailey, E., Mickelson, J., Roed, K., Lindgren, G., Von Haeringen, W., Guerin, G., Bjarnason, J., Allen, T., Binns, M. (2000). First comprehensive low-density horse linkage map based on two 3-generation, full-sibling, cross-bred horse reference families. Genomics 66, 123-134.

Swinburne, J.E., Boursnell, M., Hill, G., Pettitt, L., Allen, T., Chowdhary, B., Hasegawa, T., Kurosawa, M., Leeb, T., Mashima, S., Mickelson, J.R., Raudsepp, T., Tozaki, T., Binns, T. (2006). Single linkage group per chromosome genetic linkage map for the horse, based on two three-generation, full-sibling, crossbred horse reference families. Genomics 87, 1-29.

Trotter, G.W., McIlwraith, C.W. (1981). Osteochondrosis in horses: pathogenesis and clinical syndromes. American Association of Equine Practitioners 27, 141-160.

Van De Lest, C.H.A., Van Den Hoogen, B.M., Van Weeren, P.R., Brouwers, J.F.H., Van Golde M.L.M.G., Barneveld, A. (1999). Changes in bone morphogenic enzymes and lipid composition of equine osteochondrotic subchondral bone. Equine veterinary Journal Supplement 31, 31-37.

Van Grevenhof, E.M., Schurink, A., Ducro, B.J., van Weeren, P.R., van Tartwijk, J.M., Bijma, P., van Arendonk, J.A. (2009). Genetic variables of various manifestations of osteochondrosis and their correlations between and within joints in Dutch warmblood horses. Journal of Animal Science 87, 1906-1912.

Van Weeren, P.R. (2005). Osteochondrosis: a challenging enigma. Pferdeheilkunde 21, 285-292.

Van Weeren, P.R., Barneveld, A. (1999). The effect of exercise on the distribution and manifestation of osteochondrotic lesions in the Warmblood foal. Equine veterinary Journal, Supplement 31, 16-25.

Wade, C.M., Giulotto, E., Sigurdsson, S., Zoli, M., Gnerre, S., Imsland, F., Lear, T.L., Adelson, D.L., Bailey, E., Bellone, R.R., Blöcker, H., Distl, O., Edgar, R.C., Garber, M., Leeb, T., Mauceli, E., MacLeod, J.N., Penedo, M.C., Raison, J.M., Sharpe, T., Vogel, J., Andersson, L., Antczak, D.F., Biagi, T., Binns, M.M., Chowdhary, B.P., Coleman, S.J., Della Valle, G., Fryc, S., Guérin, G., Hasegawa, T., Hill, E.W., Jurka, J., Kiialainen, A., Lindgren, G., Liu, J., Magnani, E., Mickelson, J.R., Murray, J., Nergadze, S.G., Onofrio, R., Pedroni, S., Piras, M.F., Raudsepp, T., Rocchi, M., Røed, K.H., Ryder, O.A., Searle, S., Skow, L., Swinburne, J.E., Syvänen, A.C., Tozaki, T., Valberg, S.J., Vaudin, M., White, J.R., Zody, M.C.; Broad Institute Genome Sequencing Platform; Broad Institute Whole Genome Assembly Team, Lander, E.S., Lindblad-Toh, K. (2009). Genome sequence, comparative analysis, and population genetics of the domestic horse. Science 326 (5954), 865-867.

Willms, F., Röhe, R., Kalm, E. (1999). Genetische Analyse von Merkmalskomplexen in der Reitpferdezucht unter Berücksichtigung von Gliedmaßenveränderungen. Züchtungskunde 71, 330-345.

Winter, D., Bruns, E., Glodek, P., Hertsch, B. (1996). Genetische Disposition von Gliedmaßenerkrankungen beim Reitpferd. Züchtungskunde 68, 92-108.

Wittwer, C., Hamann, H., Rosenberger, E., Distl, O. (2006). Prevalence of osteochondrosis in the limb joints of South German Coldblood horses. Journal of Veterinary Medicine A 53, 531-539.

Wittwer, C., Hamann, H., Rosenberger, E., Distl, O. (2007a). Genetic parameters for the prevalence of osteochondrosis in the limb joints of South German Coldblood horses. Journal of Animal Breeding and Genetics 124, 302-327.

Wittwer, C., Löhring, K., Hamann, H., Distl, O. (2007b). Mapping quantitative trait loci for osteochondrosis in fetlock and hock joints and palmar/plantar osseus fragments in fetlock joints of South German Coldblood horses. Animal Genetics 38, 350-357.

Wittwer, C., Dierks, C., Hamann, H., Distl, O. (2008). Associations between candidate gene markers at a quantitative trait locus on equine chromosome 4 responsible for osteochondrosis dissecans in fetlock joints of South German Coldblood horses. Journal of Heredity 99, 125-129.

Wittwer, C., Hamann, H., Distl, O. (2009). The candidate gene XIRP2 at a quantitative gene locus on equine chromosome 18 associated with osteochondrosis in fetlock and hock joints of South German Coldblood horses. Journal of Heredity 99, 125-129.

The role of conformation on performance and predisposition to injury: is there a difference between Thorougbreds and Warmbloods

Willem Back[1] and Chris E. Kawcak[2]
[1]Department of Equine Sciences, Utrecht University, Faculty of Veterinary Medicine, 3584 CM Utrecht, the Netherlands
[2]Equine Orthopaedic Research Center, Colorado State University, Fort Collins, CO 80523, USA

The effects of conformation on lameness and athletic potential have been evaluated subjectively and are mostly based on anecdotal evidence and experience of the observer (Van Weeren and Crevier-Denoix, 2006). Some people would consider this an 'art form' in which some people have a natural talent for assessing the influence of different conformational characteristics on injury and talent. Only recently have objective conformational parameters been developed and used to assess various conformational traits on performance and injury (Back *et al.*, 1996; Holmström, 2001; Rossdale and Butterfield, 2006). The goal of this paper is to review some of the work that has been done in this area as well as emerging evidence that may lead to further objective characterization of subtle conformational traits. Within the last ten years a few classical studies have emerged relating conformational traits and injury, both for the racing Thoroughbred as well as the sporting Warmblood.

For the Thoroughbred is mainly focused on the carpus as this anatomical location is prone for injuries dealing with chip fractures as well as the fetlock for condylar fractures. Anderson and McIlwraith (2004) showed that only 5%-7% of long bone growth occurred between weaning and the 3-year-old year and therefore most bone growth is completed by a year of age. Anderson *et al.* (2004) also compared conformation to injury in Thoroughbreds. They found that carpal valgus characteristics were somewhat protective. Those horses with carpal valgus tended to have decreased carpal effusion, decreased carpal fractures, decreased carpal physeal reaction and decreased fracture incidence in the right forelimb. Those horses that were considered 'over at the knee' had increased chance of phalangeal fractures and increased fetlock physitis. Those horses with 'off-set knees' tended to have increased right front fetlock effusion and increased right front fetlock problems in general. These differences occurred even in the face of the fact that Thoroughbreds tend to have a high incidence of front fetlock problems anyway. It was also found that increased pastern length increased the chance of forelimb fracture. Therefore, today most clinicians feel that mild carpal valgus is protective and is actually normal during growth. Similar to the results of Barr (1994) they did not observe that being 'back at the knee' was an issue. However, Back *et al.* (2006) noticed in warmbloods a relationship indeed between a back at the knee conformation at square stance and carpal hyperextension at trot.

The issue of the 'normal' amount of carpal valgus was further characterized by Santschi *et al.* (2006). In this study they graded carpal and front fetlock deviations of foals, dams and sires and followed the foals from a week of age until 18 months of age. In general they found a high incidence of carpal valgus within the first week of life (94%), which decreased to roughly 21% at 18 months age. In addition, they also saw an increase in the incidence of 'off-set knees', from 8% at a week of age to upwards of 68% at 18 months of age. They also concluded that the sire phenotype was associated with the foals' carpal conformation and that the carpal valgus noticed at birth self corrects over a years period. The authors commented that it was hard to correlate the mares conformation as there is a general belief that the mares become more 'off-set' and 'toed-in' with age. They conclude that the reason for this is a change in the material properties of the bones with age and increased weight with pregnancy. They feel that most of the force is being generated medially and consequently leading to more off set knee conformation. Foals with high birth weight had an increase of 'off-set knee' conformation which they attributed to the increased weight. They also noted that foals with higher weight at birth had an increased incidence of carpal valgus conformation and a lack of selfcorrection over time. They also found that 'off-set' conformation of the carpi may have been underdiagnosed when the foals were young due to the high incidence of valgus conformation. These foals also had increase in 'toe-in' conformation which can result in increased medial limb strain (Firth *et al.*, 1998). With this information the authors further hypothesize that there may be a genetic component to the increased incidence of 'off-set' carpi and 'toed-in' conformation with increased body weight. The increased body weight is hypothesized to increase the lateral load on the distal radius and the carpus along with increased medial load on the digit and proximal metacarpal area. These offsetting forces then can lead to 'off-set knees' and inward fetlock deviation when they are very young. One contradicting observation is by Hunt (2000) where he felt that the 'off-set knees' and fetlock varus conformation usually occurs in filly's with big bodies, light bone and a wide base. He observed that this is correlated with the mares' conformation and in these cases would often recommend early weaning to reduce weight. From these studies one can conclude that the body type may dictate the physical forces transmitted through the lower limbs consequently leading to modification of the active modeling characteristics of the joints.

A recent study has shown that subtle joint shape characteristics may also lead to fracture. Kawcak *et al.* reported that racing Thoroughbreds with third metacarpal condylar fracture had significant reduction in lateral-to-medial condylar width ratio in the palmar aspect of their fractured limbs and also showed reduced lateral-to-medial condylar width ratio in the dorsal aspect of the joints in both fractured and unfractured limbs compared to horses without fracture (Kawcak *et al.*, 2009). This has led to the hypothesis that early, subtle conformational abnormalities may lead to disparity in joint shape and size, consequently predisposing some horses to fracture. With the advent of biomechanical models, including finite element modeling, further work is needed to characterize the effects of subtle abnormal forces on joint shape.

Other studies have also evaluated conformation on the incidence of injury in National Hunt racehorses (Weller *et al.*, 2006). Using 3-D motion capture Weller *et al.* found that increased intermandibular width, increased flexor angular shoulder and the increased coxal angle had a positive effect on performance. They also found that increased girth size, increased length of the hind digit and front fetlock valgus led to decrease in performance. They also found that there was an increased incidence of superficial digital flexor tendonitis with increased fetlock angle and carpal valgus and an increased incidence of pelvic fracture with increased incidence of tarsal valgus and coxal angle. The authors admitted though that this was a relatively small study with low power and that although generalizations were provided no recommendations have been made for determining at what angles breeders and trainers should select against in order to reduce injury.

Overall it appears that objective means of characterizing of conformation are needed and in the study by Santschi *et al.* (2006) the validation portion of their study showed that the coefficient of variation for subjective assessment of conformation was greater than 10%, which is well below a clinically useful tool. In that portion of the study they evaluated 48 foals over two successive days and found that 79% of the carpal grades were evaluated similarly between days and 87% of the fetlock grades were evaluated the same.

Conformation has its influence on soundness at speed performance, but also seems to have an effect in Warmbloods bred for sports performance, dressage and jumping. The majority of lamenesses are located in the distal forelimb, which is a reason in Warmbloods to have a closer look at hoof conformation in relation to performance and injuries.

Recently, the 'grassfoot' phenomenon has been unraveled, as foals with relatively longer limbs and shorter neck and head length seem to have a preference in forelimb position when grazing leading to an asymmetric development of their front feet, the so called uneven feet (Ducro *et al.*, 2009a). The steep foot is positioned backwards and the sloping foot is put forward. Warmblood studbooks tend to select their horses in not having this asymmetry. The effect of this phenomenon has been evaluated at a population level comparing studbook admission data, scoring the existence of uneven feet, with what horses have delivered in sports (Ducro *et al.*, 2009b). Length of competitive life was shorter for jumping than for dressage. A different set of risk factors was found for each level and discipline: e.g. height at withers was a risk factor at basic level in dressage and jumping, while pastern angle was a risk factor at the elite level of jumping and dressage. The trait 'uneven feet' tended to shorten the competitive life in dressage, but was a significant risk factor at the elite level of jumping.

Subjective evaluation makes statistical analysis difficult and often leads to lack of robustness in data analysis. Therefore, people have begun to develop photographic (Anderson *et al.*, 2004), videographic (Weller *et al.*, 2006) and inertial sensor technology (Barrey *et al.*, 2002) to objectively evaluate conformation. In addition, it appears that these data can be combined with joint based computer models to best evaluate the effects of conformational limb loading on the joint surfaces in the hopes of identifying morphologic characteristics that would reduce the incidence of injury.

Although reducing the incidence of injury is of great importance to the industry, these analysis techniques can be compared to performance. However, it is impossible to measure those psychological characteristics that lead to enhanced performance. It is likely that those will continue to be subjective. At this point the best that the veterinarian can do is offer counseling on the physical characteristics of an animal in order to reduce injury and possibly maximize performance potential.

References

Anderson, T.M., McIlwraith, C.W. (2004). Longitudinal development of equine conformation from weanling to age 3 years in the Thoroughbred. Eq Vet J 36, 563-570.

Anderson, T.M., McIlwraith, C.W., Douay, P. (2004). The role of conformation in musculoskeletal problems in the racing Thoroughbred. Eq Vet J 36, 571-575.

Back, W., Schamhardt, H.C., Barneveld, A. (1996). The influence of conformation on fore and hind limb kinematics of the trotting Dutch Warmblood horse. Pferdeheilkunde 12, 647-650.

Barr, A.R. (1994). Carpal conformation in relation to carpal chip fracture. Vet Rec 134, 646-650.

Barrey, E., Desliens, F., Poirel, D., *et al.* (2002). Early evaluation of dressage ability in different breeds. Eq Vet J Suppl, 319-324.

Ducro, B.J., Bovenhuis, H., Back, W. (2009a). Heritability of foot conformation and its relationship to sports performance in a Dutch Warmblood horse population. Eq Vet J 41, 139-43.

Ducro, B.J., Gorissen, B., Van Eldik, P., Back, W. (2009b). Influence of foot conformation on duration of competitive life in a Dutch Warmblood horse population. Eq Vet J 41, 144-8.

Firth, E.C., Schamhardt, H.C., Hartman, W. (1988). Measurements of bone strain in foals with altered foot balance. Am J Vet Res 49, 261-265.

Holmström, M. (2001). The effects of conformation. In: Equine Locomotion. Back W and Clayton HM, 1st edition, WB Saunders, London.
Hunt, R.J. (2000). Management of Angular Limb Deformities. In: Proc Am Assoc Equine Pract 46, 128-129.
Kawcak, C.E., Zimmerman, C.A., Easton, K.L., *et al.* (2009). Effects of Third Metacarpal Geometry on the Incidence of Condylar Fractures in Thoroughbred Racehorses 2009;197.
Rossdale, P.R., Butterfield, R.M. (2006). Conformation: a step along the pathway to objective assessment. Eq Vet J 38, 588-590.
Santschi, E.M., Leibsle, S.R., Morehead, J.P., *et al.* (2006). Carpal and fetlock conformation of the juvenile Thoroughbred from birth to yearling auction age. Eq Vet J 38, 604-609.
Van Weeren, P.R., Crevier-Denoix, N. (2006). Equine conformation: clues to performance and soundness. Eq Vet J 38, 591-596.
Weller, R., Pfau, T., Babbage, D., *et al.* (2006). Reliability of conformational measurements in the horse using a three-dimensional motion analysis system. Eq Vet J 38, 610-615.
Weller, R., Pfau, T., May, S.A., *et al.* (2006). Variation in conformation in a cohort of National Hunt racehorses. Eq Vet J 38, 616-621.

Considerations of the optimal management of horses from birth to 2 years of age

Brian D. Nielsen[1] and Chris E. Kawcak[2]
[1]Michigan State University, Department of Animal Science, East Lansing, MI 48824-1225, USA
[2]Equine Orthopaedic Research Center, Colorado State University, Fort Collins, CO 80523, USA

Trying to keep young horses sound when they enter training is a challenge faced by many trainers. Numerous factors bring rise to this challenge including things somewhat beyond the control of a trainer such as conformation. However, the management of young horses before they enter hard training is one factor that can be modified to give the greatest opportunity to prevent injuries while also optimizing the likelihood of being able to perform up to their genetic potential.

The period from birth to training is essential for laying a foundation of athletic health in the future. Although generalized health and nutrition during growth is important, the challenge in equine medicine is maximizing musculoskeletal strength in order to deal with the rigors of training. This paper is a review of general health considerations to maximize training potential in horses with an emphasis on the musculoskeletal system.

Management of young horses starts during late gestation in the broodmares. Maximal broodmare health and nutrition is essential and this nutritional management must carry on through the foal's growth period. Overall mare health and vaccination status must be optimized for the region in which the horses are housed. In addition, overall foal health must be maximized beginning with optimizing immunity.

Proper nutrition is a management issue that often does not get as much consideration as deserved. While guidelines on the nutrient requirements of young, growing horses have been reasonably well-defined (NRC, 2007), many individuals do not evaluate the rations they feed against these requirements. There are many reasons why such a ration evaluation is not performed. Obviously, not being aware of the requirements is one reason, but another reason is that the true nutrient content of the roughages and concentrates being fed are often not known. Without that knowledge, it is impossible to determine if the nutrient requirements of the animals are being met.

Even if it can be determined that nutrient requirements are being met, some equine nutritionists believe that a diet still might not be appropriate if the amount of energy in the diet is not balanced in relationship to the amount of nutrients, such as protein and minerals, that the diet contains. If excessive energy is available in relationship to the amount of nutrients that are available, poor quality growth may be the result. For instance, the animal may be gaining weight, but the ratio of body fat being deposited in relation to the amount of lean body tissue being developed may be too great. Such was the case when yearling horses were fed whole oats and hay as compared to a blended grain mix and hay (Gibbs *et al.*, 1989). Diets were isocaloric, but the oats had lower amounts of protein, Ca, and P and the end result was horses in both groups having similar weights, but the horses receiving oats instead of a balanced concentrate were shorter and fatter.

While greater fat deposition at the expense of lean tissue growth is undesirable, worse problems can develop when young horses are provided unbalanced diets. For instance, a greater incidence of dyschondroplasia was noted in foals fed a high-energy diet (Savage *et al.*, 1993). It is believed that the problem was not the result of excess energy, but due to insufficient quantities of other nutrients being consumed after horses quit eating after satisfying their demand for dietary energy. Likewise, Glade and Belling (1986) found that a high-energy diet induced osteochondrotic changes in the cartilage of weanling horses. While an attempt was made to provide a comparable increase in protein to match the increase in energy, neither calcium nor phosphorus was similarly increased resulting in a deficient nutrient to calorie ratio.

While many individuals recommend feeding a low-energy diet to avoid a rapid rate of growth, and potential developmental problems believed to be associated with fast growth, concerns about rapid growth may not be founded if the nutrient to calorie ratio is properly maintained. That being said, a recent study reported that foals having a high wither height at 30 days of age had an increased risk factor for developmental orthopaedic disease (Lepeule *et al.*, 2009). This finding could lead one to conclude that regardless of diet, horses genetically prone to rapid growth may be predisposed to growth problems. One could also question whether trying to slow growth rate is an appropriate measure. Instead, insuring a balanced ration and trying to maintain consistent growth may be more desirable.

Nutrition of foals can be managed aggressively but the biggest mistake in management is usually under-feeding due to rapid growth. A solution to this that we have employed includes monthly weighing of the foals in order to maximize nutritional benefits. Seasonal forage and ration analyses are performed, and a nutritionist is consulted. Clinical records and yearling radiographs are compared between years in order to monitor the incidence of developmental orthopedic disease as one indicator of proper nutrition.

Another interesting finding by Lepeule *et al.* (2009) was that the amount of exercise foals received was related to the incidence of developmental orthopaedic disease. Of the 292 foals in the study that received daily free exercise, only 30% were affected by osteochondrosis as compared to 53% of the 55 foals that received exercise only one to three days per week or that experienced periods with no free exercise. This agrees with work by van Weeren and Barneveld (1999), which demonstrated a trend for osteochondrotic lesions in the stifle to be less severe for foals allowed to exercise freely in pastures compared to foals kept in box stalls. These results are not surprising if one understands how the skeletal system responds to exercise.

Contrary to what most people believe, bone is a rather dynamic tissue and responds to whatever forces are applied to it (Chen *et al.*, 2010). Though it is impossible to witness with the naked eye, bone bends with applied force, such as when a horse takes a fast stride. There is a certain amount of bend that the bone 'finds desirable,' often termed the optimal strain environment (Rubin and Lanyon, 1987). When bone bends too much, the bone senses it is not strong enough and an attempt is made to lay down more bone so that when similar forces are applied, the bone will not bend as much. In contrast, if bone does not bend enough, the body senses that there is too much mineral present (which is inefficient from an energetic standpoint – carrying around more mineral than is needed will only slow a horse down when trying to escape a predator) and mineral will be lost. By losing that mineral, the bone becomes less rigid and will be able to bend more so that the optimal strain environment is once more established. Though it is not quite this simple, the phrase 'use it or lose it' typically applies to bone.

Some examples of the manifestations of bone's response to exercise, or the lack thereof, have given some pretty clear guidelines as to how bone in young horses responds to varying housing and training conditions. First, research has clearly demonstrated in numerous studies that placing young horses (weanlings, yearlings, two-year-olds) into stalls without any opportunity to sprint results in a loss of bone from the skeleton (Hiney *et al.*, 2004a; Bell *et al.*, 2001; Hoekstra *et al.*, 1999). Even walking a horse for an hour or two on a mechanical walker has been shown to be insufficient to prevent bone loss associated with stalling (Hoekstra *et al.*, 1999). And while most people would believe the galloping (cantering) done in the first few months of training would stimulate bone to become stronger, this is not the case if the horses are not given any opportunity to sprint – either forced such as when being ridden or voluntary such as when turned out (Hoekstra *et al.*, 1999). Contrary to what many would believe, research has failed to show a difference between the mineral content of two-year-olds kept on pasture and given free access to exercise versus pasture-mates that were subjected to endurance training for months in which horses were trained on a high-speed treadmill to complete 37-mile long exercise tests (Spooner *et al.*, 2008). Again, without any high-speed exercise, bone will fail to become stronger – no matter how far a horse travels in training.

Interestingly, it does not take many strides at speed to elicit a positive response. Using weanlings kept in stalls, an 80-m sprint down an alleyway once per day five times per week for a 42-day period resulted in substantially greater bone gain than was seen in similar weanlings kept in stalls without exercise (Hiney *et al.*, 2004a). There was also greater bone gain than was seen in group-housed weanlings kept in a dry-lot. And in a very dramatic response, young bull calves kept in individual stalls and that were similarly sprinted 50 meters in an alleyway of a barn five times per week showed dramatic improvements in mineral content of bone, as well as fracture force, when their bones were subjected to mechanical testing, compared to ones housed similarly but with no forced exercise and to those calves that were group-housed in a pen without exercise (Hiney *et al.*, 2004b).

The conclusions that can be drawn are simple. To gain strength necessary for activities such as racing, bone must be exposed to the large forces that accompany running at speed. Fortunately, it does not take many strides to accomplish this (and doing too many, especially when not adapted to it, certainly can cause damage). In some other species, as few as four cycles of bending (similar to a stride in the horse) have been shown to prevent disuse osteoporosis (Rubin and Lanyon, 1984). While horses do not necessarily spend a lot of time running while out on pasture, it only takes the occasional short sprint to prevent bone loss. Especially with young horses kept in a group, usually all it takes is one horse to run and then the others in the group do also. Hence, they usually sprint enough to maintain a reasonable amount of bone. Interestingly, a study conducted at Texas A&M University in the early 90's demonstrated that when yearlings were removed from pasture and placed into stalls at the onset of race training, a dramatic decrease in the mineral content of the cannon bone was observed (Nielsen *et al.*, 1997). The mineral content (and presumably bone strength) remained lower until horses began to be breezed after a few months of slow gallop training. Not surprisingly, by introducing speed when the mineral content of the cannon bone (and likely other bones) was lowest, this is when the greatest number of bone-related injuries occurred. Unfortunately, replacing mineral that was previously lost as a result of disuse is a slow process. In that study, even after racing every two weeks for nine times, the mineral content was still lower than before horses had ever entered training. Or to place the blame where it really belongs, it was still lower than before horses had ever been placed into stalls. A similar response was recently reported with young Thoroughbreds entering training and being placed into stalls in Kentucky (Pagan *et al.*, 2007).

Fortunately, if bone loss accompanying stalling occurs early in life, such bone loss can be reversed (Nielsen *et al.*, 2000). To what extent it can be reversed in older horses remains to be determined. More importantly, it is critical to remember that bone loss does not need to occur if horses are managed correctly. In a research study where yearlings were trained while on pasture, the mineral content continued to increase as would be expected with growing horses (Hoekstra *et al.*, 1999). This is in comparison to former pasture-mates that had been placed into stalls and had lost a significant amount of mineral within a month's time. Obviously, maintaining young horses on pasture at the onset of training is not practical for everyone. If such is the case, several options exist. First, a little bit of turn-out in an area that allows the horse some opportunity to run around for a short period of time is probably adequate to prevent most of the loss seen in the early stages of training. While longer periods of turn-out have advantages for a number of reasons, truthfully, if the horse is able to sprint at least 50 meters one time, that is probably sufficient for bone. If turn-out is not an option, being able to put similar short sprints on a horse being ridden can likely yield similar positive results. Granted, especially in the early stages of training, such sprints under saddle may be difficult to achieve while maintaining the proper mindset of the young athlete.

Other types of forced exercise may have advantages but have accompanying concerns. One such type of forced exercise is on a high-speed mechanical walker – often referred to as a free-flow exerciser. These walkers are a great improvement over the traditional walker because they can go faster, they allow a horse more freedom within a compartment rather than being attached by a chain, and because they usually have a much greater radius than a traditional walker. However, they are still not ideal for the prevention of bone loss. Rarely can they go as fast as one would want a young horse to sprint to experience the same load on the skeleton that would be experienced while racing. Instead, the likelihood is that lower loads would be experienced but over a greater distance. Since bone responds more to the intensity of the load, rather than the number of strides taken, this does not do one as much good as compared to a very short high-speed sprint in a straight line. Additionally, considering that the exercise in a walker is done in a circular fashion, the potential exists for cartilage damage to occur (Vernon *et al.*, 2007). Uneven loading of joints, such as going at speed through turns, can lead to early problems with osteoarthritis. Thus, one needs to be cautious about doing too much fast work in exercisers or, even worse, on a longe line. Typically, the smaller the circle and the faster the horse travels, the greater is the likelihood for damage to cartilage.

Musculoskeletal health of the foal must be addressed at birth and throughout the growth period until the start of training. This is a dynamic time for musculoskeletal growth necessitating aggressive management and examinations on a regular basis. The biggest factor in maximizing musculoskeletal health at a young age is the influence of exercise. In humans, exercise has been shown to increase bone size and density (Borer, 2005; Cooper *et al.*, 1995; Khan *et al.*, 2000). In addition, this physical activity at a young age and during maximal growth can have long lasting benefits later in life. Early exercise has also been shown to be beneficial in horses. For instance, Brama *et al.* (2009) showed that subchondral bone mineral density is significantly increased with growth and in those areas that are habitually loaded. This group also demonstrated that articular cartilage in foals is biochemically homogenous until 5 months of age and that this heterogenous appearance that occurs at 5 months of age is not only complete but can be delayed due to lack of exercise (Brama *et al.*, 2002). Articular cartilage glycosaminoglycan increases with exercise at 5 months with little change after 6 months and that there was no effect on collagen. This group further went on that stall confinement can lead to significant decreases in calcium and collagen cross link proteins in the subchondral bone (Brama *et al.*, 1999). In addition, Cornelissen *et al.* (1999) found that cross sectional area of bone increased with age but was most prominent in pasture-exercised foals compared to those that were box-rested. However, they also showed that even though box stall rest retards normal development, it can be compensated with exercise after weaning.

In a separate study, another group found that exercise can be beneficial at a young age. Using the same group of foals, several investigators found that there can be beneficial effects when exercise is supplemented to pasture activity. For instance, Dykgraaf *et al.* (2008) found a significant increase in the percentage of viable chondrocytes and an increase in Safranin O staining of articular cartilage matrix in foals that were exercised in addition to pasture turnout. In this group Moffat *et al.* (2008) also found a trend toward increase in cross sectional area of superficial digital flexor tendons in those foals that were exercised in addition to pasture turnout. Rogers *et al.* (2008a) found that supplemental exercise did not negatively affect the overall well-being of the foals and they actually found this exercise to be protective in preventing tarsocrural effusion and physeal swelling of the radius, distal third metacarpus and distal third metatarsal bones. They further went on to show that later in life those that were exercised had more pre-race training at 2- and 3-year-olds and any orthopedic problems were presented later, as opposed to earlier, compared to the pasture-reared horses (Rogers *et al.*, 2008b). In addition, Kawcak *et al.* (2000) found at 18 months of age that those foals that had early exercise had increased bone formation rate and increased subchondral bone in some areas of the distal third metacarpal condyle but that they also had significant decrease in glycosaminoglycan staining in some areas of articular cartilage. The superficial digital flexor tendon is not biochemical homogenous at birth like articular cartilage but does functionally adapt over time (Lin *et al.*, 2005). Therefore, one can conclude that overall early exercise is beneficial although care must be taken in not over-stressing these foals.

To further elaborate on the latter point, we have seen some foals develop subchondral cystic lesions during development which may be attributed to trauma to the subchondral bone plate as demonstrated by Ray *et al.* (1996). This point has been further elaborated on in humans by Naughton *et al.* (2000) who found that, in humans, those children undergoing rapid growth and increased training had overuse injuries. In addition, Parfitt (1994) showed that rapid growth in children can actually lead to increased cortical porosity and susceptibility to fracture. Therefore, the amount of exercise that foals and young horses undergo should be managed aggressively in order to prevent over exercising.

Musculoskeletal management of foals occurs starting at birth. The maturity of the foal can be variable due to gestational age and the amount of exercise dictated by the physical maturity of the foal. Those foals that are subjectively deemed to be relatively immature will be confined to a small stall and then expanded to a larger stall and a small run over approximately a week depending on their level of immaturity. They will then get limited amounts of turnout which will be built up over time until the foals are turned out full-time. The general health must also be taken into consideration. The mare's health is also important during this time as ailments can lead to confinement of the foal. With hospitalized mares, if it is possible these mares and foals are usually taken outside twice a day and, with mare held in hand, the foals are allowed to exercise around a paddock. This limited amount of stimulation often times will be enough to maintain the strength of the musculoskeletal system.

Angular limb deformities are a significant problem in foals and take an aggressive management scheme to manage appropriately. Some angular limb deformities will correct on their own and some deformities are actually normal at birth. For instance, newborn foals are normally born with 4 to 5 degrees of valgus conformation to their knees which corrects on its own with broadening of the chest. Therefore, mistakes can be made in trying to correct this angular limb deformity at this early age. Some minor angular limb deformities will also correct with exercise, foot manipulation and some have reported improvement with splinting. Regardless of the location and severity of angular limb deformity, the ultimate goal is to get the foals some form of turnout as soon as possible. We typically start with 1 to 2 hours of turnout a day and have the farm managers monitor the limbs closely. If the angular limb deformity worsens at the end of turnout, then we ask that they restrict the amount of turnout even further. If, for instance, the foals come in with slightly worse contracture of the joints, then again the turnout is limited and gradually built up. Conformation will change dramatically during growth. For instance, a foal with a narrow chest will start to expand and grow rapidly throughout the growth period and so early assessment of conformation, although critical, should be considered in light of how it will change later in life. In addition, it is good to monitor the mentality of these foals earlier in life as this may be a predictive indicator of performance later in life.

Many musculoskeletal changes occur at weaning. As Brama *et al.* (2002) showed, heterogenous changes to articular cartilage biochemical configurations will be complete at approximately 5 months of age. They also found that lack of bone formation early in life due to restrictive exercise can be compensated after 5 months. In addition, Moffat *et al.* (2008) found that cross sectional area of the superficial digital flexor tendon will be maximized between 5 and 8 months of age. Therefore, exercise is essential during the weaning period in order to maximize soft tissue integrity. One concern during weaning is the stress that the foals undergo during this time period. We have subjectively seen that some foals undergo mild respiratory illness during this time, supposedly due to the increased stress. We have seen a reduction in vitamin K status in the foals during this time which may have a modest effect on bone formation. The key, though, is to continue to allow the weanlings to exercise during this time period. Another beneficial effect of turnout is farm managers and breeders can get a subjective assessment of the individuals at this time. The maturity and aggressiveness can be monitored and give some insight as to performance selection in the future.

As yearlings, continual turnout is maintained and radiographs are typically taken sometime during the yearling year. The types of radiographs taken are discipline specific (Contino *et al.*, 2009; Kane *et al.*, 2003a,b). The influence of sales preparation in some breeds is slightly concerning. In order to maximize muscular appearance, some foals undergo underwater and over ground treadmill exercise, which may or may not be beneficial. Kawcak *et al.* (2000) found that over ground treadmill exercise can have some positive and negative effects on articular cartilage in bone. In addition, nutrition seems to be modified during this time in order to maximize growth and weight gain, which may have an influence on musculoskeletal integrity. During the yearling year, these horses again are monitored for lameness and any mild changes are addressed diagnostically in an aggressive fashion.

In preparation for breaking and training, physical examinations are essential. This is similar to what is done in the human field where pre-season physical examinations are not only key to identifying potential problems, but are now mandatory in most collegiate sports. During the early training period it is also essential to monitor these horses to ensure that they are indeed tolerating the early training period.

While there are many factors that go into the proper development of a young equine athlete, two that demand attention are nutrition and exercise. Unfortunately, many individuals do not evaluate their nutritional programs adequately to ensure they are providing the proper nutrients. Even more unfortunate is the failure of many individuals to allow young horses to experience the correct type of exercise needed to maximize skeletal strength. The most important item to remember is that short sprints are critical for optimal bone development. Whether the sprints are forced or occur when horses are allowed free exercise is not critical. However, exercise that involves substantial turning should be avoided.

In summary, management of horses from birth to 2-years of age is a dynamic process. Although a conservative approach to managing musculoskeletal problems is essential, sometimes aggressive changes in management are needed in order to maximize musculoskeletal growth and integrity. Therefore, young horses that are intended for an athletic future should be monitored on a regular basis and changes in management considered if high incidence of problems result.

References

Bell, R.A., Nielsen, B.D., Waite, K., Rosenstein, D., Orth, M. (2001). Daily access to pasture turnout prevents loss of mineral in the third metacarpus of Arabian weanlings. J. Anim. Sci. 79:1142-1150.

Borer, K.T., 2005. Physical activity in the prevention and amelioration of osteoporosis in women: interaction of mechanical, hormonal and dietary factors. Sports Med. 35:779-830.

Brama, P.A., Firth, E.C., Van Weeren, P.R., Tuukkanen, J., Holopainen, J., Helminen, H.J., Hyttinen, M.M. (2009). Influence of intensity and changes of physical activity on bone mineral density of immature equine subchondral bone. Equine Vet. J. 41:564-571.

Brama, P.A., TeKoppele, J.M., Bank, R.A., Van Weeren, P.R., Barneveld, A. (2002). Development of biochemical heterogeneity of articular cartilage: influences of age and exercise. Equine Vet. J. 34:265-269.

Brama, P.A., TeKoppele, J.M., Bank, R.A., Van Weeren, P.R., Barneveld, A. (1999). Influence of different exercise levels and age on the biochemical characteristics of immature equine articular cartilage. Equine Vet. J. Suppl. 31:55-61.

Chen, J.H., Liu, C., You, L., Simmons, C.A. (2010). Boning up on Wolff's Law: mechanical regulation of the cells that make and maintain bone. J. Biomech. 43(1):108-118.

Contino, E.K., McIlwraith, C.W., Park, R.D. (2009). Prevalence of radiographic changes in yearling and 2-year-old Quarter Horses. Am. Assoc. Equine Pract. Pp. 470.

Cooper, C., Cawley, M., Bhalla, A. *et al.* (1995). Childhood growth, physical activity, and peak bone mass in women. J. Bone Miner. Res. 10:940-947.

Cornelissen, B.P., Van Weeren, P.R., Ederveen, A.G., Barneveld, A. (1999). Influence of exercise on bone mineral density of immature cortical and trabecular bone of the equine metacarpus and proximal sesamoid bone. Equine Vet. J. Suppl. 31:79-85.

Dykgraaf, S., Firth, E.C., Rogers, C.W., Kawcak, C.E. (2008). Effects of exercise on chondrocyte viability and subchondral bone sclerosis in the distal third metacarpal and metatarsal bones of young horses. Vet. J. 178:53-61.

Gibbs, P.G., Sigler, S.H., Goehring, T.B. (1989). Influence of diet on growth and development of yearling horses. J. Equine Vet. Sci. 9(4):215-218.

Glade, M.J., Belling, T.H. (1986). A dietary etiology for osteochondrosis. J. Equine Vet. Sci. 6:151-155.

Hiney, K.M., Nielsen B.D., Rosenstein, D.S. (2004). Short-duration exercise and confinement alters bone mineral content and shape in weanling horses. J. Anim. Sci. 82(8):2313-2320.

Hiney, K.M., Nielsen, B.D., Rosenstein, D., Orth, M.W., Marks, B.P. (2004). High-intensity exercise of short duration alters bovine bone density and shape. J. Anim. Sci. 82:1612-1620.

Kawcak, C.E., McIlwraith, C.W., Norrdin, RW, Park, R.D., Steyn, P.S. (2000). Clinical effects of exercise on subchondral bone of carpal and metacarpophalangeal joints in horses. Am. J. Vet. Res. 61:1252-1258.

Hoekstra, K.E., Nielsen, B.D., Orth, M.W., Rosenstein, D.S., Schott, H.C., Shelle, J.E. (1999). Comparison of bone mineral content and bone metabolism in stall- versus pasture-reared horses. Equine Vet. J. Suppl. 30:601-604.

Kane, A.J., Park, R.D., McIlwraith, C.W., Rantanen, N.W., Morehead, J.P., Bramlage, L.R. (2003a). Radiographic changes in Thoroughbred yearlings. Part 1: Prevalence at the time of the yearling sales. Equine Vet. J. 35:354-365

Kane, A.J., McIlwraith, C.W., Park, R.D., Rantanen, N.W., Morehead, J.P., Bramlage, L.R. (2003b). Radiographic changes in Thoroughbred yearlings. Part 2: Associations with racing performance. Equine Vet. J. 35:366-374.

Khan, K., McKay, H.A., Haapasalo, H. *et al.* (2000). Does childhood and adolescence provide a unique opportunity for exercise to strengthen the skeleton? J. Sci. Med. Sport 3:150-164.

Lepeule, J., Bareille, N., Robert, C., Ezanno, P., Valette, J.P., Jacquet, S., Blanchard, G., Denoix, J.M., Seegers, H. (2009). Association of growth, feeding practices and exercise conditions with the prevalence of Developmental Orthopaedic Disease in limbs of French foals at weaning. Prev. Vet. Med. 89:167-177.

Lin, Y.L., Brama, P.A., Kiers, G.H., De Groot, J., Van Weeren, P.R. (2005). Functional adaptation through changes in regional biochemical characteristics during maturation of equine superficial digital flexor tendons. Am. J. Vet. Res. 66:1623-1629.

Moffat, P.A., Firth, E.C., Rogers, C.W., Smith, R.K., Barneveld, A., Goodship, A.E., Kawcak, C.E., McIlwraith, C.W., Van Weeren, P.R. (2008). The influence of exercise during growth on ultrasonographic parameters of the superficial digital flexor tendon of young Thoroughbred horses. Equine Vet. J. 40:136-140.

Naughton, G., Farpour-Lambert, N.J., Carlson, J., Bradney, M., Van Praagh, E. (2000). Physiological issues surrounding the performance of adolescent athletes. Sports Med. 30:309-325.

Nielsen, B.D., Potter, G.D., Morris, E.L., Odom, T.W., Senor, D.M., Reynolds, J.A., Smith, W.B., Martin, M.T. (1997). Changes in the third metacarpal bone and frequency of bone injuries in young Quarter Horses during race training -- observations and theoretical considerations. J. Equine Vet. Sci. 17(10):541-549.

Nielsen, B.D., Waite, K.L., Bell, R.A., Rosenstein, D.S. (2000). Long-term pasture housing promotes bone mineral deposition in the third metacarpus of previously stalled weanlings. The Elite Show Jumper. Conf. Equine Sports Med. Sci. 2000. pg. 157-159.

NRC (2007). Nutrient requirements of Horses. 6th rev. ed. Natl. Acad. Press, Washington, DC.

Pagan, J.D., Lawrence, L.A., Nash, D. (2007). Skeletal adaptations with the onset of training in thoroughbreds. Proc. 20th Symp. Equine Sci. Soc. pp. 148-149.

Parfitt, A.M. (1994). The two faces of growth: benefits and risks to bone integrity. Osteoporos. Int. 4:382-398.

Ray, C.S., Baxter, G.M., McIlwraith, C.W. (1996). Development of subchondral cystic lesions after articular cartilage and subchondral bone damage in young horses. Equine Vet. J. 28:225-232.

Rogers, C.W., Firth, E.C., McIlwraith, C.W., Barneveld, A., Goodship, A.E., Kawcak, C.E., Smith, R.K., Van Weeren, P.R. (2008a). Evaluation of a new strategy to modulate skeletal development in Thoroughbred performance horses by imposing track-based exercise during growth. Equine Vet. J. 40:111-118.

Rogers, C.W., Firth, E.C., McIlwraith, C.W., Barneveld, A., Goodship, A.E., Kawcak, C.E., Smith, R.K., Van Weeren, P.R. (2008b). Evaluation of a new strategy to modulate skeletal development in racehorses by imposing track-based exercise during growth: the effects on 2- and 3-year-old racing careers. Equine Vet. J. 40:119-127.

Rubin, C.T., Lanyon, L.E. (1984). Regulation of bone formation by applied dynamic loads. J. Bone Joint Surg. Am. 66(3):397-402.

Rubin, C.T., Lanyon, L.E., 1987. Osteoregulatory nature of mechanical stimuli: function as a determinant for adaptive remodeling in bone. J. Orthop. Res. 5(2):300-310.

Savage, C.J., McCarthy, R.N., Jeffcott, L.B. (1993). Effects of dietary energy and protein on induction of dyschondroplasia in foals. Equine Vet. J. 16:74-79.

Spooner, H.S., Nielsen, B.D., Woodward, A.D., Rosenstein, D.S., Harris, P.A. (2008). Endurance training has little impact on mineral content of the third metacarpus in two-year-old Arabian horses. J. Equine Vet. Sci. 28:359-362.

Van Weeren, P.R., Barneveld, A. (1999). The effect of exercise on the distribution and manifestation of osteochondrotic lesions in the Warmblood foal. Equine Vet. J. Suppl. 31:16-25.

Vernon, K.L., Riggs, L., Ellis, S., Coverdale, J.A., Gibbons, J. (2007). A sheep model: the effects of circular and linear exercise on macroscopic changes in articular cartilage. Proc. 20th Symp. Equine Sci. Soc. pp. 91-92.

An investigation into the effect of exercise history on the osteochondral unit in the equine distal tarsal joints

Caroline A. Tranquille[1], Rachel C. Murray[1], Sue J. Dyson[1], Tony S. Blunden[1], Tim D.H. Parkin[2] and Allen Goodship[3]
[1]Centre for Equine Studies, The Animal Health Trust, Lanwades Park, Kentford, Newmarket, Suffolk CB8 7UU, United Kingdom
[2]Institute of Comparative Medicine, Faculty of Veterinary Medicine, University of Glasgow, Glasgow G61 1QH, United Kingdom
[3]The Royal Veterinary College and Institute of Orthopaedics and Musculoskeletal Science, UCL, Hertfordshire AL9 7TA, United Kingdom

Take home message

Ridden exercise influences cartilage and subchondral bone thickness and the severity of lesions in the osteochondral unit in the equine distal tarsal joints. Sites that are predisposed to osteoarthritis (OA) appear to be more affected than sites not predisposed to OA.

Introduction

Distal tarsal pain is a common cause of hind limb lameness that affects horses from a variety of breeds and exercise histories (Bohanon, 1997). Distal tarsal joint OA is a major cause of hock pain, but disease development is poorly understood. To improve the understanding of OA development, we need to understand normal tarsal structure and function. Loading is associated with an increase in subchondral bone (SCB) thickness, leading to site-specific variations in thickness, as a response to site specific variations in load intensity (Oettmeier *et al.*, 1992; Firth *et al.*, 1999; Murray *et al.*, 2001). It is important to understand normal patterns of SCB thickness in order to understand the development of osteochondral pathology. Intersite variation in SCB structure may be a result of differences in anatomical location and subsequent differences in loading (Milz *et al.*, 1997; Brama *et al.*, 2002). In the equine carpus, osteochondral morphology and mechanical properties were influenced by location within a joint, and by exercise intensity (Murray *et al.*, 1999).

The distal tarsus is under constant compressive forces, with greater load on the dorsal and lateral aspects (Schamhardt *et al.*, 1989). A repeatable pattern of SCB thickness across the distal tarsus has been seen in mature horses with no history of hind limb lameness. This may reflect adaptation of bone to site-specific mechanical loading, but it is not known when this pattern develops (Branch *et al.*, 2005).

It is important to understand normal variations in the equine distal tarsal osteochondral unit in association with exercise in order to establish how pathological changes occur.

Hypotheses

1. Ridden exercise is associated with increased cartilage and subchondral bone thickness, especially at sites predisposed to OA.
2. Ridden exercise is associated with an increase in number, and severity, of lesions in the osteochondral unit.

Material and methods

Thirty cadaver tarsi from horses without lameness that had undergone pasture-exercise only (Group P, n=10), low-intensity general purpose exercise (Group L, n=10) and elite level competition (Group E, n=10) were used. Selected sites from the centrodistal (CD) and tarsometatarsal (TMT) joints underwent histological preparation. Articular cartilage (AC), hyaline cartilage (HC), calcified cartilage (CC) and SCB thickness were measured at standard sites. Exercise groups were compared using a one-way ANOVA or Mann-Whitney U test at a significance level of $P<0.05$.

The same sections were graded histologically using an adapted grading system (Yagi *et al.*, 2005; Kim *et al.*, 2003) to describe location, depth and shape of lesions, cellular arrangement, organisation at the cartilage and SCB margins and organisation of the SCB. A larger score signified more severe pathological change. Exercise groups were compared using descriptive statistics.

Results

Group E AC was thicker at all sites, with a statistically significant difference at the lateral proximal aspect of the third metatarsal bone (MT3) ($P=0.024$). There were no significant differences between groups in HC thickness. CC was thicker at all sites in Group E, with a statistically significant difference at the lateral proximal aspect of MT3 ($P=0.019$). Mediolateral and proximodistal patterns of AC and CC thickness were different between groups.

In the CD joint, lesions were present in Groups L and E, and positioned only on the medial aspect. The cellular arrangement was consistent between the 3 groups with a higher score at a dorsomedial location. Groups L and E had higher scores than Group P for the organisation of the margins and SCB, with higher scores at the dorsomedial location. In the TMT joint, lesions were seen across the whole joint surface with more severe lesions at the lateral location in all 3 groups.

Overall, Group E had higher scores for cellular arrangement, margin and SCB organisation. In all 3 groups, greater scores were seen at a dorsolateral location.

Discussion

Results from this study supported our hypotheses. In general, the overall thickness of the cartilage and SCB was lowest in Group P horses, slightly greater in Group L horses, and maximal in Group E horses. Thicknesses were greatest at sites predisposed to OA.

Increased HC thickness with exercise is reported to occur in immature joints of horses (Murray *et al.*, 1999; Firth and Rogers, 2005; Martinelli *et al.*, 2002), dogs (Oettmeier *et al.*, 1992) and humans (Jones *et al.*, 2003). Greater CC thickness with exercise has been reported in immature joints of horses (Murray *et al.*, 1999) and dogs (Oettmeier *et al.*, 1992) undergoing treadmill exercise. It has been suggested that variations in loading across the articular surface are reflected by local variations in CC thickness (Murray *et al.*, 1999; Martinelli *et al.*, 2002; Müller-Gerbl *et al.*, 1987). Findings in our study revealed corresponding increases in all the tissues of the mature osteochondral unit in a non-interventional over-ground (and not treadmill) situation. Ridden general purpose and competition horses are not ridden or trained until skeletal maturity, so it is likely that increase cartilage thickness was induced by functional adaptation after maturity.

SCB thickness increased with increased exercise intensity, which supports findings in other equine studies (Murray *et al.*, 2001; Firth and Rogers, 2005; Branch *et al.*, 2005; Firth *et al.*, 1999; Norrdin *et al.*, 1998) and those in others species (Oettmeier *et al.*, 1992; Radin *et al.*, 1982). Small numbers of high strains stimulate bone remodeling (Lanyon, 1992; Marcus, 1996); elite competition exercise could be associated with greater SCB thickness. Some sites from Group P tarsi had thicker SCB than tarsi from Group L horses. It is possible that there was residual SCB thickness from a previous period in which Group P horses had raced at 2 years of age. This suggests that SCB thickness is retained over a period of at least 9 years without changing. Alternatively, the thicker SCB in some sites of tarsi from Group P horses, compared with tarsi from Group L horses, which could be related to different types of activities undertaken by the 2 groups. At pasture, exercise is self-controlled and generally consists of continual low strains interspersed with short periods of high strains over variable terrain or as horses run and twist, which could stimulate bone remodeling (Lanyon, 1992). Low-intensity exercise on soft, consistent training surfaces is more likely to induce consistent low-to-moderate strains in the distal tarsal joints. Previously, it has been shown that different exercise types are associated with different SCB thickness patterns across the distal tarsal articular surfaces, likely reflecting different loading patterns sustained by the different types of exercise undertaken (Murray *et al.*, 2007). These horses are also often restricted to stables for a portion of the day in contrast to continual movement at pasture. If tarsi from horses that only had pasture exercise, and not previously raced, had been used then SCB thickness may have been different.

In this study, dorsomedial lesions were seen in the CD joint and dorsolateral lesions were seen in the TMT joint, which may reflect this pattern of loading across the distal tarsal joints. The dorsal changes that have been detected may be due to dorsal compression that the joint experiences while the horse is jumping or performing dressage movements. A medial to lateral load transfer has previously been described (Schamhardt *et al.*, 1989) and supported by bone modelling assessed using nuclear scintigraphy in horses with a history of no hindlimb lameness (Murray *et al.*, 2004).

The kissing 'cavitation and hillock' lesion was most frequently seen in Groups L and E. This may be related to the rotational loading experienced at these sites (Lanovaz *et al.*, 2002) which could reflect the type of defect seen. This lesion type could be associated with the turning and circles that ridden horses perform, which may accentuate the rotational movement within the distal tarsal joints (Branch *et al.*, 2005; Murray *et al.*, 2007).

SCB histologic morphology was normal in all 3 exercise groups, except at the dorsomedial aspect of the CD and dorsolateral aspect of the TMT joints. Radiographic and histologic changes with respect to age in the CD joint of Icelandic ponies (Bjornsdottir *et al.*, 2004) and Thoroughbred horses (Laverty *et al.*, 1991) have been described. In Icelandic ponies, SCB sclerosis was not a primary factor in the development of OA. It was thought to be caused by uneven distribution of load throughout the joint. In Thoroughbred horses, changes in the SCB plate, joint junctions and sclerotic SCB increased in severity with increasing age. The aetiopathogenesis of OA is not fully understood, however the differences between the 2 breeds may be because of differences in type and intensity of work and that OA is hereditary in the Icelandic pony (Bjornsdottir *et al.*, 2000).

Lesions and higher histopathological scores were correlated with ridden exercise. It is possible that this is related to carrying the extra weight of the rider or because of altered loading patterns, such as specific dressage movements (passage or piaffe) or jumping (Peham *et al.*, 2004). These factors mean that the tarsus is under more frequent intense loading, or compression, for a greater proportion of each stride (Holmstrom and Drevemo, 1997; Van Den Bogert *et al.*, 1994) and that this could lead to more histopathological changes.

Conclusions

Ridden exercise influences AC, CC, HC and SCB thickness and the severity of lesions and histological features in the osteochondral unit in the equine distal tarsal joints. Sites that are predisposed to OA are more affected than sites not predisposed to OA.

References

Bjornsdottir, S., Arnason, Th., Axelsson, M., *et al.*, (2000). The heritability of degenerative joint disease in the distal tarsal joints in Icelandic horses. Livest. Prod. Sci, 63:77-83.

Björnsdóttir, S., Ekman, S., Lord, P. (2004). High detail radiography and histology of the central intertarsal joint of young Icelandic horses. Equine Vet J. 36: 5-11.

Bohanon, T.C. (1997). Pain associated with the distal tarsal joints of the hock. In: Current therapy in equine medicine 4. Robinson NE, ed. Philadelphia: WB Saunders Co, pp 88-93.

Brama, P.A.J., Tekoppele, J.M., Bank, R.A., Barneveld, A., Van Weeren, P.R. (2002). Biochemical development of subchondral bone from birth until age eleven months and the influence of physical activity. Equine Vet J. 34: 143-149.

Branch, M.V., Murray, R.C., Dyson, S.J., Goodship, A.E. (2005). Is there a characteristic distal tarsal subchondral bone plate thickness pattern in horses with no history of hind limb lameness? Equine Vet J. 37: 450-455.

Firth, E.C., Delahunt, H., Witchel, J.W., Birch, H.L., Goodship, A.E. (1999). Galloping exercise induces regional changes in bone density within the third and radial carpal bones of Thoroughbred horses. Equine Vet J. 31: 111-115.

Firth, E.C., Rogers, C.W. (2005)Musculoskeletal responses of 2-year-old Thoroughbred horses to early training. 7. Bone and articular cartilage response in the carpus. N Z Vet J 53:113-122.

Holmstrom, M., Drevemo, S. (1997). Effects of trot quality and collection on the angular velocity in the hindlimbs of riding horses. Equine vet. J. Suppl. 23 62-65.

Jones, G., Bennell, K., Cicuttini, F.M. (2003)Effect of physical activity on cartilage development in healthy kids. Br J Sports Med 37:382-383.

Kim, D.Y., Taylor, H.W., Moore, R.M., Paulsen, D.B., Cho, D.Y. (2003). Articular chondrocyte apoptosis in equine osteoarthritis. The Vet J 166: 52-57.

Lanovaz, J.L., Khumsap, S., Clayton, H.M., Stick, J.A., Brown, J. (2002) Three-dimensional kinematics of the tarsal joint at the trot. Equine Vet J. Suppl 34: 308-313.

Lanyon, L.E. (1992). Control of bone architecture by functional load bearing. J Bone Miner Res 7:369-375.

Laverty, S., Stover, S.M., Belanger, D., O'Brien, T.R., Pool, R.R., Pascoe, J.R., Taylor, K., Harrington, T. (1991) Radiographic, high detail radiographic and histological findings of the distal portion of the tarsus in weanling, young and adult horses. Equine Vet J. 123: 413-421.

Marcus, R. (1996). Mechanisms of exercise effects on bone. In: Bilezikian JP, Raisz LG, Rodan GA, eds. Principles of bone biology. Academic Press Inc, pp 1135-1146.

Martinelli, M.J., Eurell, J., Les, C.M., Fyhrie, D., Bennett, D. (2002). Age-related morphometry of equine calcified cartilage. Equine Vet J 34: 274-278.

Milz, S., Eckstein, F., Putz, R. (1997). Thickness distribution of the subchondral mineralisation zone of the trochlear notch and its correlation with the cartilage thickness: An expression of functional adaptation to mechanical stress acting on the humeroulnar joint? Anat Rec. 248: 189-197.

Müller-Gerbl, M., Schulte, E., Putz, R. (19870. The thickness of the calcified layer of articular cartilage: a function of load supported? J Anat 154: 103-111.

Murray, R.C., Whitton, R.C., Vedi, S., Goodship, A.E., Lekeux, P. (1999). The effect of training on the calcified zone of equine middle carpal articular cartilage. Equine Vet J. Suppl 30: 274-278.

Murray, R.C., Vedi, S., Birch, H.L., Lakhani, K.H., Goodship, A.E. (2001). Subchondral bone thickness, hardness and remodelling are influenced by short-term exercise in a site-specific manner. J Orthop Res. 19: 1035-1042.

Murray, R.C., Dyson, S.J., Weekes, J., Branch, M.V., Hladick, S. (2004). Nuclear scintigraphic evaluation of the distal tarsal region in normal horses. Vet Radiol Ultrasound. 45: 345-351.

Murray, R., Branch, M., Dyson, S., Parkin, T., Goodship, A. (2007). How does exercise intensity and type affect equine distal tarsal subchondral bone thickness? J. Appl. Phys. 102: 2194-2200.

Norrdin, R.W., Kawcak, C.E., Capwell, B.A., McIlwraith, C.W. (1998). Subchondral bone failure in an equine model of overload arthrosis. Bone. 22: 133-139.

Oettmeier, R., Arokoski, J., Roth, A.J., Helminen, H.J., Tammi, M., Abendroth, K. (1992). Quantitative study of articular cartilage and subchondral bone remodelling in the knee joint of dogs after strenuous running training. Bone Miner Res. Suppl 2: 419-424.

Peham, C., Licka, T., Schobesberger, H., Meschan, E. (2004). Influence of the rider on the variability of the equine gait. Hum Mov Sci, 23: 663-671.

Radin, E.L., Orr, R.B., Kelman, J.L., Paul, I.L., Rose, R.M. (1982) Effect of prolonged walking on concrete on the knees of sheep. J Biomech 15: 487-492.

Schamhardt, H.C., Hartman, W., Lammertink, J.L.M.A. (1989). Forces loading the tarsal joint in the hind limb of the horse, determined from in vivo strain measurements of the third metatarsal bone. Am J Vet Res. 50: 728-733.

Van Den Bogert, A.J., Jansen, M.O., Deuel, N.R. (1994). Kinematics of the hind limb push-off in elite show jumping horses. Equine vet. J., Suppl. 17: 80-86.

Yagi, R., McBurney, D., Laverty, D., Weiner, S., Horton Jr., W.E. (2005). Intrajoint comparisons of gene expression patterns in human osteoarthritis suggest a change in chondrocyte phenotype. J Orthop Res 23: 1128-1138.

Training strategies and days lost to injury vary in Swedish showjumping yards

Cecilia Lönnell, Lars Roepstorff, Elin Hernlund, Caroline Schöön and Agneta Egenvall
The Swedish College of Agricultural Sciences, Uppsala, Sweden

Take home message

Intensity and volume of training and risk of injury vary between Swedish showjumping riders riding at S-level.

Introduction

Lameness is the most common diagnosis in equine veterinary practice (Clausen *et al.*, 1990; Kaneene *et al.*, 1997; Penell *et al.*, 2005; Egenvall 2006). Studies in racehorses have demonstrated that the risk of orthopaedic injury varied between trainers and with training strategies and use of surfaces (Rossdale 1985; Moyer and Fisher 1992; Estberg *et al.*, 1996; 1998; Boston 2000; Parkin 2005; Verheyen *et al.*, 2005; 2006; Cogger *et al.*, 2006). Very little has been published in relation to injuries affecting horses involved in equestrian sports. No such studies have been conducted in showjumpers. We hypothesised that, as has been previously shown in racehorses, training strategies and injury risk vary at herd level.

Material and methods

We conducted a prospective pilot field study during April-October 2009 in Sweden. Riders recruited were 17 professional/full time showjumping riders ranked in country's Top 100 in 2008, starting at S level in 2008, and 2 showjumping riders at S-/professional level outside the Top 100 with minimum 3 horses in training.

Participating riders kept a standardised daily training diary with time and intensity of flat work, fitness work, jumping and hacking and use of riding surfaces, non-ridden activities, including pasture time, plus health data for horses (n=144). Fourteen yards or equestrian centres were included (eight riders used equestrian centres with shared arenas). At baseline participating riders and the visiting researcher (CL) made arena surface evaluations based on seven criteria: surface firmness, dampening, permanent vs elastic deformation, grip, evenness and uniformity and total impression. Riders also used roads, forest tracks/paths and grass as riding surfaces. All horses were European Warmbloods, aged 4-18, competing from Novice to 5* International level. Riders were asked to exclude horses in the yard not expected to stay the full six months. Thus not all horses in all yards were included (also due to time restraints as some riders had up to 18 horses in training). The Swedish study was part of an international collaborative epidemiological and biomechanical project on show jumping training and surfaces with elite and amateur riders in Sweden, the Netherlands, Switzerland, the UK and Denmark.

Results (preliminary)

Training strategies, including intensity and type of training, varied between riders. Differences included the emphasis on flatwork (min 1.5 - max 7 sessions a week, median 3), hacking (0-6 sessions a week, median 1.8). For jumping and fitness work the number of sessions varied from 0 to 2 sessions a week. Speed of canter/gallop work varied from 350 to 800 meters/minute. Strategies of jumping sessions also varied between riders, from mainly grid work /low fences to full courses with competition height. Estimated subjective intensity of sessions varied from 5% (hacking at walk) to 85% (fitness gallop).

Preliminary analysis of prospective training protocol data from May and June showed that the mean time recorded for each session of fitness (gallop or hill climbing), flatwork, hacking and jumping was extremely similar, ~40 minutes and varied only little by rider. However the cumulative time varied significantly, as a mean for each riders horses over the two months. The analysis were based on horses with a maximum of three days lost to training over the period and deemed to be in full work. For hacking the cumulative mean minutes per horse over two months varied between riders from 0 to 2,480 minutes, for fitness between 0 and 1,655 minutes, for flatwork from 370 to 2,330 minutes and for jumping from 0 to 1,535 minutes

Total daily time outside the stable (including ridden work and non-ridden activities, i.e. pasture time, walker, treadmill and/or lungeing) varied from 1.8 to 6.5 hours. Indoor and outdoor arena surfaces used included sand, sand plus fibre or sand plus woodchip. Arena surfaces used differed not only in composition of material but also age and standard of maintenance.

Prospectively, the incidence of orthopaedic injury in horses in the study varied by rider from between 0-100%. The 100% rate was for all horses included in the study (n=8) in one yard. For all cases in the study diagnosis were made by an equine veterinarian, chiropractor, or blacksmith in the case of hoof abscesses. The riders' protocol information on diagnosis was confirmed and clarified by telephone with the person responsible.

Conclusions

This study demonstrates that strategies for training of showjumpers including intensity, and risk of injury, vary between riders at top level. Further analysis of data and research will clarify possible associations between training factors and risk of injury in showjumpers. Based on early results the study confirms the hypothesis of variations in risk of injury with different training strategies. Early analysis and subjective observations do not support surface as a lone risk factor of injury, for surfaces used under normal training conditions, but training, surface and competition strategies as joint influences.

References

Boston, R.C., Nunamaker, D.M. (2000). Gait and speed as exercise components of risk factors associated with onset of fatigue injury of the third metacarpal bone in 2-year-old Thoroughbred racehorses. Am J Vet Res 61, 602-607.

Clausen, *et al.* (1990). Analysis of disease data in the German warmblood. Zuchtungkd 62, 167-178.

Cogger, N., Perkins, N., Hodgson, D.R., Reid, S.W., Evans, D.L. (2006). Risk factors for musculoskeletal injuries in 2-year-old Thoroughbred racehorses. Prev Vet Med 74, 36-43.

Egenvall, A., Penell, J.C., Bonnett, B.N., Olson, P., Pringle, J. (2006). Mortality of Swedish horses with complete life insurance between 1997 and 2000: variations with sex, age, breed and diagnosis. Vet Rec 158, 397-406.

Estberg, L., Gardner, I.A., Stover, S.M., Johnston, B.J. (1998). A case-crossover study of intensive racing and training schedules and risk of catastrophic muscoloskeletal injury and lay-up in California Thoroughbred racehorses. Prev Vet Med 33, 159-170.

Estberg, L., Stover, S.M., Gardner, I.A., Drake, C.M., Gohnson, B., Ardans, A. (1996). High-speed exercise history and catastrophic racing fracture in Thoroughbreds. Am J Vet Res 57, 1549-1555.

Kaneene, J.B., Ross, W.A., Miller, R. (1997). The Michigan equine monitoring system. 2. Frequencies and impact of selected health problems. Prev Vet Med 29, 277-292.

Moyer, W., Fisher, J.R.S. (1992). Bucked shins, effects of differing track surfaces and proposed training regimens. Proc 37th Annual Convention of AAEP. Pp 541-546.

Parkin, T.D., Clegg, P.D., French, N.P., Proudman, C.J., Riggs, C.M., Singer, E.R., Webbon, P.M., Morgan, K.L. (2005). Risk factors for fatal lateral condylar fracture of the third metacarpus/metatarsus in UK racing. Eq Vet J 37, 192-199.

Penell, J.C., Egenvall, A., Bonnett, B.N., Olson, P., Pringle, J. (2005). Specific causes of morbidity among Swedish horses insured for veterinary care between 1997 and 2000. Vet Rec 157, 470-477.

Rossdale, P.D., Hopes, R., Wingfield, Digby, N.J., Offord, K. (1985). Epidemiological study of wastage among racehorses 1982 and 1983. Vet Rec 116, 66-69.

Verheyen, K.L., Henley, W.E., Price, J.S., Wood, J.L. (2005). Training-related factors associated with dorsometacarpal disease in young Thoroughbred racehorses in the UK. Eq Vet J 37, 442-448.

Verheyen, K., Price, J., Lanyon, L., Wood, J. (2006). Exercise distance and speed affect the risk of fracture in racehorses. Bone 39, 1322-1330.

The role of the shoes in performance and injury prevention; what´s in for the (proned to) navicular lame horse

J. Thomason[1] *and W. Back*[2]

[1]*Department of Biomedical Sciences, Ontario Veterinary College, University of Guelph, Ontario, Canada*

[2]*Department of Surgery and Anaesthesiology of the Domestic Animals, Faculty of Veterinary Medicine, Ghent University, Merelbeke, Belgium*

Abstract

By parsing out the stance into its kinematically and kinetically important phases, it is possible to separate the significance of each to the varied activities required of performance horses and the kinds of injury they might experience. This approach also leads to a critique of the effects of shoes on the mechanics of each stage.

Introduction

The primary roles of shoes in performance horses on arena surfaces is to provide support (e.g. hoofwall) and traction (e.g. through caulks and rims), but at which stages do these functions most likely are to cause injury? Our approach is, first, to separate the stance into its biomechanically distinct stages – primary and secondary impact, support, rollover and toe-off – and to describe the mechanical features of each. Where possible, experimental data are used, but it is necessary to resort to basic principles in many cases. We discuss the types of injury that may be associated with each stage of the stance during each activity, and this component is largely based on reasoned speculation. Incorporated in this discussion is the role of shoeing in modifying performance or possibly causing or preventing injury. One objective of this exercise is to give the practitioner a guide that may assist in predicting the effects of preventive or therapeutic measures for some foot and limb injuries. The other is to show how much of the discussion and questions raised await future research for verification, clarification or definitive answers.

Most of the stages of the stance have been described in primary literature (Hjertén and Drevemo, 1994) and reviews (Back and Clayton, 2001; Johnston and Back, 2006; Thomason and Peterson, 2008). Here we separate the support stage into loading, midstance, and unloading.

Primary impact

As the hoof meets the ground it decelerates rapidly to zero velocity (within 1-3 milliseconds on a firm surface), primarily in a vertical direction. The shock of impact is heavily damped by the soft tissues of the hoof (with the assistance of the ground surface if it has the appropriate cushion) (Gustås *et al.*, 2001). Forces on the foot are relatively low, because only the mass of the hoof and pasterns participates in this collision. In the equation $F = ma$, the acceleration a may exceed 500g at high speed on a hard surface (Gustås *et al.*, 2006). By keeping mass m low – it is effectively only the mass of the digit – force F is also usually kept within the limits of strength of the bones and soft tissues of the hoof and limb.

Role in injury

In sports performance Warmbloods, it is likely that this stage has a minor role in injury, because the landing velocities of the hoof are lower than for fast locomotor performance as in Thoroughbreds. At slower speeds the concussion shock of impact is reduced, thus any injuries that do occur, would largely be to tissues close to the hoof capsule itself (e.g. bruising of the lamina f.e. on uneven sand & stone track).

Effect of different activities

The magnitude of the shock on impact will certainly vary between front and hind feet, and lead or non-lead. There is also good evidence from high-speed videos that the four feet are loaded differently on landing from a jump (Schamhardt *et al.*, 1993). But this variability is unlikely to affect the role of primary impact in injury, because the shock associated with it probably falls within a low range of magnitudes. The exception might be landing from a jump. In this case, the effective mass in the equation $F = ma$ could include a portion of the mass of the whole body, because of the downward trajectory of its centre of mass. In this case, the low acceleration would tend to counterbalance the higher mass to keep forces on the limb within tolerable limits.

Effect of shoes

Sports performance horses generally work on compliant surfaces, which will cushion the shock of primary impact. Certainly metal shoes will transmit the shock to the foot, and oscillate at its own natural frequency on impact (modulated by contact with both the surface and the hoof, Back *et al.*, 2006). The shock-damping and absorbing properties of the surface, coupled with the presumed low magnitudes, are likely to override any effect of the shoe during this brief stage of the stance. The navicular lame horse should be shod with a shoe with insoles and pad to damping these oscillations.

Secondary impact

As soon as the hoof is at rest on the surface, the body of the horse – which is still moving forward – collides with its own implanted and stationary leg (Ruina *et al.,* 2005). The body tends to push the leg forwards, forcing the hoof to slide and then stop (Pardoe *et al.*, 2001; Vos and Riemersma, 2006). In return, the leg tends to retard or brake the motion of the body, resulting in a caudally directed horizontal component (Fh) of ground reaction force. This component oscillates during secondary impact then shows a negative peak towards the end of this stage, which seems to differ between fore and hind limbs (Back *et al.*, 1995).

Role in injury

Secondary impact has the potential to have a large role in causing injury. During the normal slide-stop action of the hoof that occurs in this stage, the coffin bone may be forced forward, compressing the laminar junction between itself and the capsule. This action is certainly plausible, though has not been conclusively demonstrated.

If the foot slips forward, this action has the possibility of forcing the digital flexor muscles into rapid, unpredicted eccentric contraction, which can cause tears within a muscle. If the foot comes to too rapid a halt, it would exacerbate any forward motion of the coffin bone, as described in the preceding paragraph. Of possible greater consequence, shortening the duration of the slide will increase the magnitude of the horizontal component (Fh) of the ground reaction force, exerting larger-than-normal bending moments on the cannon bone (Pratt, 1997). Even small increments in moment would induce large stresses in long bones such as the cannon bone.

In practice, more consideration is given to the effects of traction aids on propulsion, that is, as an aid to performance. Their effects on secondary impact are at least if not more important in the context of injury prevention. It may be that a single traction device on the shoe may not be sufficient, and that separate ones for secondary impact and propulsion (to be discussed below) should be developed.

Effect of different activities

Landing from a jump is likely to be the activity most affected by variation in the duration of secondary impact. If traction is too low or high, the resulting slippage or grabbing of the foot, respectively, will almost certainly increase the risk of injury, owing to the forward and downward momentum of the horse, which increases the effective mass on the foot during this stage (Vos and Riemersma, 2006).

Effect of shoes

Traction between the shoe and the surface is important during this stage, in all activities, to control the duration of the phase and distance moved during the slide-stop motion. In this context, 'traction' is a complex concept, involving the ratio of the vertical and horizontal components of the ground reaction force (vertical force = Fv, and horizontal force = Fh), the frictional coefficient between the material of the shoe and that of the surface, the ability of the surface material to resist shear, the cross-sectional shape of the shoe, and the effect of traction devices attached to the shoe. In principle, it should be possible to perform experiments and tests to link the surface properties and the force ratios in a specific activity to the effect of a specific grab or caulk added to the shoe. The process would require standardised testing of surfaces and the effects of shoes and traction devices. If a range of such data were collected, it would be possible to generate a table to indicate which shoes and grab types were most appropriate for a given set of field conditions (Vos and Riemersma, 2006). Such a table would be produced with the aim of prescribing the best traction device to aid performance without raising the risk of injury; in racehorses traction devices like toe grabs, seem to increase the risk of catastrophic limb failures (Kane *et al.*, 1996). When extreme braking force are applied f.e. a rubber shoe, the acute sliding seems to be mostly compensated at the fetlock area resulting in diffuse swelling.

Support: loading

This stage overlaps with primary and secondary impact, as forces begin to act between the hoof and ground from the moment of their contact. By the end of secondary impact, loading is well underway: vertical force (Fv) on the foot has risen to approximately 40% of its peak (during steady-speed locomotion). Fv continues to rise during the loading phase, peaking approximately at midstance. The horizontal (braking) force (Fh) peaks at the end of secondary impact, then becomes progressively less to reach zero at midstance (during steady-speed locomotion). When the animal is accelerating from a start, Fh reaches zero before midstance, and does not reach zero until after midstance when the animal is slowing to a stop.

Role in injury

There are no data on the role of this stage of the stance in causing injury. But there is certainly great potential for injury during the stage, for two reasons: one is the rate at which loading is increasing, and the other is the changing ratio of Fv to Fh. Many biological tissues are sensitive to the rate in which large loads are applied: the faster, the more dangerous. The ratio of Fv to Fh is significant for a reason introduced under secondary impact: this ratio, in combination with the orientation of the leg, determines the bending moments exerted by the ground reaction forces on the long bones of the limb. Even small increments in moment induce large stresses in long bones such as the cannon bone and radius.

Effect of different activities

Taking off for a jump will certainly affect the rate of loading on the hindlimb, and landing will have its effect on the front limbs. Turning and cutting activities will also be significant, because they introduce a new force component to the discussion: a horizontal, transversely directed component, Ft, which is perpendicular to the craniocaudal component Fh. For a cutting motion, the force Ft is dependent on the acceleration of the center of mass of the whole body in a lateromedial direction. For turning, Ft is generated by the centrifugal force on the body and its equal-and-opposite centripetal component of the ground reaction force. Its magnitude is dependent on the body mass, the instantaneous velocity, and the radius of the turn. Without banking of the surface, Ft can induce lateromedial bending moments on the long bones, and unevenly applied pressures on the surfaces of the joints and its collateral ligaments. Owing to the lever arm provided by the digit about the fulcrum of the fetlock, Ft will exert torque about the long axis of the cannon bone and radius.

Effect of shoes

During steady-state locomotion in a straight line, the effect of shoes is essentially limited to one contentious question: does the shoe limit the expansion of the hoof, and thereby inhibit presumed beneficial effects of that expansion? There are no definitive data to answer that question. Data from strain gauges indicate subtle changes in how the hoof expands, but no significant restriction in the degree of expansion (Thomason, 1998). Data from wires stretched around the heels, show some reduction of heel expansion (Roepstorff *et al.*, 2001), but the pliability of the heels does not allow the inference that motion was similarly restricted at the quarters.

In a turn or cutting motion, the effect of shoes is to provide traction to prevent the hoof from slipping owing to force Ft, which is likely to increase rapidly throughout the loading stage. If the ratio of Ft to Fv falls below the coefficient of friction then slippage will occur. A traction aid, by digging into the surface, will bring the shear resistance of the surface in to the equation. It is less likely that the negative effects of traction aids, as were described for secondary impact, are significant during the loading stage. The foot is planted during loading, and the purpose of shoes it to keep it planted, not to bring it to a stop as in secondary impact.

Support: midstance

The few milliseconds either side of midstance comprise the most important stage in supporting the bodyweight of the animal, because this is when the vertical component of ground reaction force (Fv) is at its peak. On the forefeet, that peak may exceed body weight at a slow trot, and exceed twice body weight at a gallop, or when landing from a jump. It is generally lower on the hind feet by between 20 and 30% (Back *et al.*, 2006).

Role in injury

The sheer magnitude of the forces on the foot midstance implicate this stage very strongly in causing traumatic bone fractures, and tendon and ligament ruptures or strains. Chronic joint problems will certainly be exacerbated if not initiated by joint loadings at this time.

Extension of the fetlock, which reaches its full excursion at midstance, is extremely important in reducing the peak magnitude of Fv, and in storing recoverable energy in the suspensory apparatus. The trade-off for these advantages is that Fv has considerable mechanical advantage, resulting in forces on the suspensory apparatus and cannon bone that theoretically exceed Fv by a factor of 2 or more. If the resultant force from Fv and Fh is not closely aligned with the axis of the cannon bone, it will exert considerable moments on the bone, which is vulnerable to bending as previously mentioned.

In the hind leg, the considerable torque about the hock from the large muscles that act through the calcaneal tendon (e.g. the gastrocnemius, biceps femoris and semitendinosus), is responsible for pressures on the many articular facets within the hock joint. The magnitude and distribution of these pressures is a prime suspect for chronic joint injury.

Effect of different activities

Taking off for a jump puts the hindlimb bones at risk, but probably not the hoof itself. The action requires sufficient force to propel the mass of the animal vertically. Stresses in the tibia and metatarsus are correspondingly elevated; even over low jumps (0.75m), stresses may reach more than double the value for a medium-fast trot, and approaching 50% of the maximum stress that bone material can withstand (Biewener *et al.*, 1988).

Landing from a jump induces stresses in the metacarpus and radius of equivalent to those experienced by the hindlimb bones on take off (Biewener *et al.*, 1983). Of greater concern is that the stresses in the metacarpus become less predictable, because the direction of the bending moment varies. Peak force on the hoof also equal or exceed those at fast gaits, suggesting that the hoof may be vulnerable to injury from them.

Turning or cutting motions are accompanied by the same issues as described for the loading stage – the effects of bending moments from Ft on long bones of the limb – perhaps exacerbated as loading reaches its peak.

Effect of shoes

The points raised under loading also apply for midstance.

Support: unloading

This stage extends from midstance until the hoof leaves the ground. In its latter stages it is accompanied by the rolling motion of the hoof from the ground and breakover. Vertical force Fv on the foot reduces from its peak at midstance to zero once contact with the ground is broken, following a line that is a very close approximation to a sinusoidal waveform.

While Fv falls rapidly during the unloading stage, horizontal force Fh increases from zero near midstance (in the steady state) to peak near the midpoint of unloading. It then decreases towards toe off. Unloading is, therefore, the primary propulsive stage of the stance. Generation of Fh is primarily from the hind legs (Back *et al.*, 1995).

Role in injury

Unloading should usually be less significant for injury than midstance, because force magnitudes are generally falling, but there are some important exceptions to this statement. Rollover provides one exception (and will be discussed below), as does acceleration from a start, because of the high bending forces on the metatarsus and tibia during acceleration. Slipping of the foot if traction is lost is also a probable cause of soft-tissue injury, for reasons similar to those discussed under secondary impact.

Effect of different activities

Any activity that requires propulsion will have a strong component of Fh during this stage, including taking off from a jump, accelerating from a start.

Effect of shoes

The most important effect of shoes in this stage is providing traction. Traction is not aided by the fact that Fv is falling while Fh is reaching its propulsive peak during the stage. Once the ratio of Fh:Fv falls below the coefficient of friction of the hoof on surface, then the foot will slip. Traction aids dig into the surface to enlist the help of the shear resistance of the surface material (Zebarth and Sheard, 1988). The navicular lame horse shod with a so called eggbar shoes will thus experience less slipage, but the centre of pressure is shifted more towards the heels (Rogers and Back, 2003).

Rollover and toe-off

This stage is the last phase of unloading, beginning as soon as the heels leave the surface. Both Fv and Fh are falling from 30-50% of their peak values towards zero at toe off. The hoof itself unrolls then pushes off from the ground.

Role in injury

This stage is important in that altering its duration strongly affects the kinematics of the limb during the swing phase, which in turn affects the kinetics of the next stance. Forcing a shorter or longer stance, under those performance activities which induce higher loading conditions, will affect the forces and stresses acting on bones and soft tissues. If more muscular control is necessary to perform the activity, muscular fatigue may become a factor in injury. If breakover and toe-off are delayed, residual tension in the deep and superficial digital flexor tendons may flick the foot back sufficiently fast that rate-dependent injury to those tendons is possible. This speculative suggestion is supported by work that shows higher magnitudes of acceleration of the hoof after toe off in galloping Thoroughbreds than the decelerations on impact with the surface (Schaer *et al.*, 2006).

Rollover is strongly implicated as a cause of injury to soft tissues within the hoof. Even though the forces on the foot are falling rapidly to zero, they become concentrated at the toe as soon as the heels begin to lift. Strain gauges at the toe show a marked spike at rollover that may exceed the magnitude of peak strain which occur just after midstance. Essentially the force is tending to peel off the toe of the hoof from the bearing surface upwards. In a healthy horse, this tendency is resisted by the laminar junction, but it is likely that some laminar bruising occurs in log-toed feet as a result of the peeling action. In a hoof with chronic laminitis, laminae at the toe are vulnerable to separation at this stage to a greater extent than any other component of the stance. If the hoof has white line disease, separation of sole and wall at the toe during rollover is a threat if the white line is sufficiently compromised.

Effect of different activities

Action of the limb will certainly affect the mechanics of rollover, as in extended or collected gaits, or exaggerated kinematics of the limb. It is difficult to predict, without experimental data, exactly what these effects will be.

Effect of shoes

Two components of shoe design are important for this stage: the shape of the cross-section at the toe and the presence and location of traction aids. Evidence is beginning to accumulate that a rolled toe is beneficial in many circumstances for preventing the delay of toe off, and reducing loading on the toe during rollover (Van Heel *et al.*, 2006). There is a generally held idea that traction is necessary at the toe to maximise propulsion, perhaps as the toe is forced into the ground when the heels lift. But by this point, most of the propulsive impulse from Fh has been generated earlier in the unloading stage. A small amount of traction at the toe may be necessary to prevent the foot slipping out and affecting the timing of the swing, but traction to assist propulsion is mostly unnecessary at this time. On the basis of this observation, traction aids at or just behind the point of breakover on the shoe might be more beneficial than at the toe. It would be interesting to test this hypothesis, as no relevant data seem to exist at present. The navicular lame horse seems to be helped by so called rolled shoes that provide a lower so called indicative moment around the navicular/coffin (Van Heel *et al.*, 2006).

The swing phase

The effect of shoeing on the swing phase cannot be ignored because of the principle of the moment of inertia, which is captured in the aphorism 'a pound on the foot is worth ten on the back'. The effort required to swing a heavy shoe can rapidly fatigue a performing horse, as well as give it considerable problems controlling the lateromedial oscillations of its limbs. The effect of shoe weight on kinematics of the swing has similar implications for risk of injury as delay of breakover.

Concluding remarks

Let us take as a goal the elimination, or at least a dramatic reduction in the frequency of foot and limb injuries of direct biomechanical cause in performance horses (and other elite equine athletes). Information for this purpose that is currently available to practitioners involved with such animals is largely empirical, based on years of accumulated observation and experience. The purpose of this paper was to approach a description of the scope of the task from the perspective of available biomechanical research data. By describing the scope, in terms of the mechanical stages of the stance and their effect on performance and injury, we hope to show how much of it is being addressed by current research, and how much remains to be done. For the practitioner, it is hoped that there are a few nuggets of information in this paper that may influence how you think about the causes of mechanical injuries. But our intent was to provide a conceptual rather than pragmatic framework for working towards the goal of reducing injuries. Recent progress allows us a modicum of hope that the goal is not an unreachable Holy Grail, but is indeed attainable within a foreseeable period of time.

References

Back, W. (2001) The role of the hoof and shoeing. In: Back W, Clayton HM (2001) Equine locomotion, 1st Edition, W.B. Saunders, London. Pp. 135-166.

Back, W., Schamhardt HC, Hartman W, Barneveld A (1995) Kinematic differences between the distal portions of the forelimbs and hind limbs of horses at the trot. Am J Vet Res 56, 1522-1528.

Back, W., Van Schie, M.H.M., Pol, J.N. (2006) Synthetic shoes attenuate hoof-impact in the trotting warmblood horse. Eq Comp Exerc Phys 3, 143-151.

Biewener, A.A., Thomason, J., Lanyon, L.E. (1983) Mechanics of locomotion and jumping in the forelimb of the horse (Equus): in vivo stress developed in the radius and metacarpus. J Zool, London 201, 67-82.

Biewener, A.A., Thomason, J.J., Lanyon, L.E. (1988) Mechanics of locomotion and jumping in the horse (Equus): in vivo stress in the tibia and metatarsus. J Zool, London 214, 547-565.

Gustås, P., Johnston, C., Hedenström, U., Roepstorf, L., Drevemo, S. (2006) A field study on hoof deceleration at impact in Standardbred trotters at various speeds. Eq Comp Exerc Physiol 3, 161-168.

Gustås, P., Johnston, C., Roepstorff, L., Drevemo, S. (2001) *In vivo* transmission of impact shock waves in the distal forelimb of the horse. Eq Vet J Suppl, 11-15.

Hjertén, G., Drevemo, S. (1994) Semiquantitative analysis of hoof-strike in the horse. J Biomech 27, 997.

Johnston, C., Back, W. (2006) Hoof ground interaction: when biomechanical stimuli challenge the tissues of the distal limb. Eq Vet J 38, 634.

Kane, A.J., Stover, S.M., Gardner, I.A., Case, J.T., Johnson, B.J., Read, D.H., Ardans, A.A. (1996) Horseshoe characteristics as possible risk factors for fatal musculoskeletal injury of thoroughbred racehorses. Am J Vet Res 57, 1147-1152.

Pardoe, C.H., McGuigan, M.P., Rogers, K.M., Rowe, L.L., Wilson, A.M. (2001) The effect of shoe material on the kinetics and kinematics of foot slip at impact on concrete. Eq Vet J Suppl 33, 70-73.

Pratt, G.W. (1997) Model for injury to the foreleg of the Thoroughbred racehorse. Eq Vet J Suppl, 30-32.

Roepstorff, L., Johnston, C., Drevemo, S. (2001) In vivo and in vitro heel expansion in relation to shoeing and frog pressure. Eq Vet J 33, 54-57.

Rogers, C.W., Back, W. (2003) Wedge and eggbar shoes change the pressure distribution under the hoof of the forelimb in the square standing horse. J Eq Vet Sci 23, 306-309.

Ruina, A,, Bertram, J.E.A., Srinivasan, M. (2005) A collisional model of the energetic cost of support work qualitatively explains leg sequencing in walking and galloping, pseudo-elastic leg behavior in running and the walk-to-run transition. J theoretical biol 237, 170.

Schaer, B.L.D., Ryan, C.T., Boston, R.C., Nunamaker, D.M. (2006) The horse-racetrack interface: a preliminary study on the effect of shoeing on impact trauma using a novel wireless data acquisition system. Eq Vet J 38, 664-670.

Thomason, J.J. (1998) Variation in surface strain on the equine hoof wall at the midstep with shoeing, gait, substrate, direction of travel, and hoof shape. Eq Vet J Suppl, 86.

Thomason, J.J., Peterson, M.L. (2008) Biomechanical and mechanical investigations of the hoof-track interface in racing horses. Vet Clin N Am. Eq. Pract. 24, 53-77.

Van Heel, M.C.V., Van Weeren, P.R., Back, W. (2006) Shoeing sound warmblood horses with a rolled toe optimises hoof-unrollment and lowers peak loading during breakover. Eq Vet J 38, 258-262.

Vos, N.J., Riemersma, D.J. (2006) Determination of coefficient of friction between the equine foot and different ground surfaces: an in vitro study. Eq Comp Exerc Phys 3, 191-198.

Zebarth, R.J., Sheard, R.W. (1988) Impact and shear resistance of turf grass racing surfaces for Thoroughbreds. Am J Vet Res 46, 778-784.

On track diagnosis of upper airways obstructions that cause reduced performance in racehorses (trotters) and their treatment

A. Ekfalk
Solvalla, Equine Respiratory Clinic, Stockholm, Sweden

Introduction

The upper airway has a complex physiologic function. The most important of several functions is to be a conduit for air to and from the lungs, and because the horse is an obligate nasal breather, a normal upper airway is critical in this species. For example, the equine upper airway has a large dead space volume, high resistance to airflow, and it tends to collapse in response to negative pressures generated during inspiration. For these reasons, the upper airway may well be a limiting factor in the horse´s exercise capacity, and tolerances in the upper airways are minimal.

A normal horse at rest breathing 15 times a minute with a tidal volume of 5 l has a minute ventilation of 75 l. During exercise respiratory rate and tidal volume increase to achieve a minute ventilation of approximately 1,500 l.

Thus, if the function of the upper airways as a conduit for airflow is used to the maximum during exercise in normal horses, it is easy to understand that small upper airway lesions can significantly impact upper airway function during exercise and further affect performance.

Respiratory surgery is currently receiving a bad press. Results are not really satisfactory because the diagnosis is too often made at rest, it is therefore often incorrect and the proposed surgery often fails.

Examination

History

Before beginning the examination, a complete history of the horse should be obtained. Specific questions should be asked about respiratory noise, exercise intolerance, coughing, nasal discharge and any previous treatment or surgery.

Physical examination

The physical examination begins with a visual inspection of the horse, his general health, muscles, presence of any nasal or ocular discharge and lymphoid tissue.

Video-endoscopy

Video-endoscopic examination at rest is still the primary diagnostic tool. A lot of diagnosis can be obtained from a complete resting endoscopic examination. The patient should not be sedated and should be restrained only with a twitch to ensure no interference with the assessment of airway function.

The normal pharynx of an adult horse shows a light red colour, has no lymphoid hyperplasia, the epiglottis should always be positioned dorsal to the palate and should have a distinct edge with a clear vascular pattern on the dorsal surface. The arytenoid cartilage should be evaluated for their overall appearance, relative position and degree of movement.

Video-endoscopic Examination during Exercise

Although a great deal of information can be gained from endoscopy in the resting horse, there are many occasions when a functional abnormality is suspected but no abnormalities are detected during the resting endoscopy examination.

Treadmill endoscopy

Treadmill endoscopy was until 2008 the easiest and most reliable way to make a diagnosis, but this examination must also be evaluated critically. The exercising conditions are not the same on the treadmill compared to examination on the racetrack. We must consider the reins, position of the head and neck, weight of the driver, ground conditions and the high speed which often is necessary to discover dysfunction in the upper airway. Horses also need a schooling and testing period on the treadmill before it is possible to do the examination.

Overground Exercise Endoscopy

In 2008 we started to use the DRS Dynamic Respiratory Scope for the OEE (Overground Exercise Endoscopy). This video-endoscope is designed to enable respiratory endoscopies to be performed during exercise. The examinations can be done under normal working conditions, similar to a race.

The DRS consists of Video-endoscope, Light source-battery processor, Transmitting-recording device, and a Receptor (monitor-screen). After the video-endoscopy at rest has been performed the horse is taken out to the track for warming up, approx. 3- 4,000 m. After this the DRS is positioned on the horse.

The DRS endoscope is installed in one of the horse´s nostrils (usually the left one). The endoscope is strapped to a special DRS bridle. The transmitter/processor is attached to the horse. The examination is displayed on the receiver in real time. Using the remote control, the veterinary assistant can start the recording remotely. At the end of examination, the recorded images are downloaded to a computer and examination can be shown to the trainer/owner on a wide screen.

The examinations are performed at the Equine Respiratory Clinic, at Solvalla Race track. Since January 2009 until March 2010 we have examined about 240 horses.

Pathological findings and their treatment

Dorsal Displacement of the Soft Palate (DDSP)

Dysfunction of the pharyngeal branch of the vagus nerve associated with inflammatory disease in the guttural pouch can interfere with some muscles in this area and lead to DDSP. This condition is a dynamic condition. The soft palate displaces over the epiglottis mostly during intensive exercise. The horse produces an expiratory noise, but OEE has shown us that the obstruction is more extensive during inspiration. The condition leads to bad performance the last 500m in the race.

Treatment: The horse should be at least 3 years old before I recommend surgical options. Laryngeal Tie Forward Technique (LTFT) is the one that we use nowadays. A success rate of 80-82% has been shown by Woodie *et al.* (2005).

Laryngeal Hemiplegia (LH)

Left recurrent laryngeal hemiplegia is characterized by paresis or paralysis of the left arytenoids cartilage and vocal fold. It manifests clinically as exercise intolerance and inspiratory respiratory noise ('roaring') during exercise. Right-sided hemiplegia and bilateral arytenoids dysfunction are uncommon.

Treatment: 'Tie Back' surgery can stabilize the affected side of the larynx during inspiration and prevent dynamic collapse of the airway during exercise. Laryngeal ventriculectomy may improve airflow and reduce the 'roaring' sound during exercise.

Epiglottic Retro Flexion (ERF)

Epiglottic retro flexion is a common cause of exercise intolerance. There are usually no respiratory noises in this condition. Epiglottis tends to raise and cause an occlusion for the airflow into the trachea. It is sometimes possible to see a tendency of retro flexion with the video-endoscope, but the diagnose will be established with OEE/DRS.

Treatment: Surgical correction of the soft palate 'staphylectomy' and myotomy of M. Sternothyroideus in both sides of thyroid cartilage.

Epiglottis Entrapment (EE)

Epiglottic entrapment is a less common cause of respiratory noise and exercise intolerance. In this condition, the aryepiglottic fold completely envelops the apex and lateral margins of the epiglottis. The distinct margins of the epiglottis and the dorsal epiglottic vascular pattern are obscured by a fold of aryepiglottic mucosa. Clinical signs of epiglottic entrapment include inspiratory and expiratory respiratory noise during exercise and poor exercise performance. Some affected horses can race successfully with the condition.

Treatment: Surgical correction by laryngotomy where the fold over the epiglottis is removed.

Axial Deviation of Aryepiglottic Folds (ADAF)

This is an uncommon condition that causes bad performance in racehorses. Diagnosis of ADAF can only be made by video-endoscope during high-speed exercise. Collapse of the aryepiglottic folds, usually the left one cause an obstruction of the airflow.

Treatment: Transendoscopic laser excision of the aryepiglottic folds can be performed safely in standing horses.

Study by Axel Wallman. Examensarbete 2010:26

The study included 110 warm blooded trotters that have been examined for abnormal noise, poor performance or both. The horses were examined with endoscopy, both during rest and maximum exercise. The findings were then compared with each other. Diagnostic images were obtained from all the horses. Thus, the prevalence can be assessed for the examined population. The examinations have all gone well without incidents or danger for the horses, equipment or personnel.

Table 1. Diagnosis by OEE/DRS.

	Abnormal noise	Poor performance	Both	Total	
	N	N	N	N	%
DDSP	5	11	20	36	33
LH	1	7	3	11	10
ERF	1	6	2	9	8
ADAF	0	2	4	6	5
Normal	7	37	4	48	44
Total	14	63	33	110	100

Table 2. Endoscopy at rest compared with OEE/DRS.

Endoscopy at rest	N	Diagnosis OEE / DRS							
		DDSP	LH II	LH III	LH IV	LH sin/dx	ERF	ADAF	Normal
Normal	88	33	0	3	0	0	5	6	41
ERF	9	1	0	0	0	0	4	0	4
LH II	8	1	2	3	1	0	0	0	2
LH III	4	0	0	0	3	1	0	0	0

Summary

56% of the examined horses showed some kind of obstruction in the upper airways and 44% were normal. The most common cause of obstruction was DDSP. 88 horses were without signs of obstruction when they were examined at rest but 53% of these horses showed obstruction when they were examined by OEE/DRS. 17 horses were suspected to have obstruction problems at rest but 6 of them were totally normal when examined with OEE/DRS.

It is therefore important to do OEE/DRS to have a better diagnosis to do an adequate treatment and improve success rate. Equally important it is not to do surgery in those horses that do not have an upper airway problem!

References

Auer, J.A., Stick, J.A. (2006) Equine Surgery. Third edition.

Pollock, P.J., Reardon, R.J.M., Parkin, T.D.H., Johnston, M.S., Tate, J., Love, S. (2009) Dynamic respiratory endoscopy in 67 Thoroughbred racehorses training under normal ridden exercise conditions Eq Vet J 41, 354-360.
Desmaizieres, L.-M., Serraud, N., Plainfosse, B., Michel, A., Tamzali, Y. (2009) Dynamic respiratory endoscopy without treadmill in 68 performance Standardbred, Thoroughbred and saddle horses under natural training conditions. Eq Vet J 41, 347-352.
Woodie, J.B., Ducharme, N.G., Kanter, P., Erb, H.N. (2005) Surgical advancement of the larynx (laryngeal tie forward) as a treatment for dorsal displacement of the soft palate in horses. A prospective study 2001-2004. Eq Vet J 37, 418-423.

Comparison of cytological profiles of bronchoalveolar lavage fluid – BALF - obtained from left and right lungs according to conditions of conservation and preparation

Valérie Deniau[1,4], Laetitia Jaillardon[2], Guillaume Fortier[3] and Anne Couroucé-Malblanc[1]
[1]Clinique Equine, Ecole Nationale Vétérinaire, Agroalimentaire et de l'alimentation de Nantes-Atlantique, Atlanpôle - La Chantrerie BP40307, 44307 Nantes cedex 3, France
[2]Laboratoire Des Dosages Hormonaux, ONIRIS, Ecole Nationale Vétérinaire, Agroalimentaire et de l'alimentation de Nantes-Atlantique, Atlanpôle - La Chantrerie BP40307, 44307 Nantes cedex 3, France
[3]Laboratoire Frank Duncombe, 1 route de Rosel, 14053 Caen cedex, France
[4]Clinique vétérinaire, Domaine de Grosbois, 94470 Boissy Saint Léger, France

Take Home Message

There is no significant difference of the cytological profile of BALF obtained from right or left lung in the same horse. However, when considering a cellular profile with more than 10% neutrophiles as diagnostic criteria for the presence of Inflammatory Airway Disease (IAD), the final interpretation of the BALF cytology may differ in some horses in relation with the side of the sample. Also, the conditions of conservation, the technique of preparation and lecture may influence the percentage of neutrophiles.

Introduction

Cytology of bronchoalveolar lavage fluid (BALF) is a widely used diagnostic technique for evaluation of the lower respiratory tract in sport and racehorses. Percentage of neutrophils, eosinophils, mast cells and haemosiderophages are the main results taken in consideration for the diagnosis of Inflammatory Airway Disease (IAD) or Exercise Induced Pulmonary Haemorrhage (EIPH) (Couetil and Denicola, 1999; Couetil *et al.*, 2007). However, variations between methods of sampling, conditions of conservation, techniques of preparation and lecture may be of concern when interpreting results.

Couetil and Denicola (1999) have demonstrated differences in neutrophils percentages between pre- and post-exercise BALF in racehorses. Also, the effect of the volume of fluid infused has been studied by Sweeney *et al.* (1992).

Pickles *et al.* (2002c) evaluated the effects of time, temperature and of two different fixatives on equine BALF cytology. They showed that the time taken for a significant reduction in total nucleated cell count (TCC) and cell viability of unfixed BALF samples decreased as the storage temperature increased. Also, alterations in cells morphology was observed when unfixed BALF samples were conserved 48h at 4 °C, 24h at 18 °C and 8h at 38 °C (Pickles *et al.*, 2002) respectively.

Although a BAL can be performed via a gastroscope (Waldridge and Welles, 2006), in practice it is mainly done with a cuffed tube without visualization of the lower airways (Mansmann and King, 1998). It is known that blind positioning of the BAL tube leads to the right lung in a majority of cases. However, questions remain about the possible differences between the right and the left lung.

The aims of this study were to compare cytological profiles of BALF obtained from left and right lungs in the same horse, and to evaluate the effects of time, temperature and laboratory techniques on these profiles.

Material and methods

Seven adult horses, two males and five mares, age 4 to 17 years, were included in this study. Two successive BAL were performed at rest using a 9 mm silicone cuffed tube (Bivona). Prior to manipulation the horses were sedated with a combination of romifidine (35 μg/kg BWT IV) and butorphanol (0.2 mg/kg BWT IV).

The first BAL was performed in a classical 'blind' technique. The cuffed tube was passed via the ventral nasal meatus into the lower airways until it could not be further advanced. Once the tube was wedged in a bronchus, the distal cuff was inflated with 5 ml of air to form a seal with the bronchus and 120 ml sterile saline were infused in one time, and immediately aspirated. The volume of fluid retrieved was recorded. However, it has been previously demonstrated that even if BALF retrieved volume is very low, cytological analysis of samples can be of diagnostic value (Pickles *et al.*, 2002a).

The cuff was deflated and, before the tube was removed, an endoscope was introduced in the trachea up to the carina in order to visualize in which main bronchus the tube was positioned. Under endoscopic guidance the tube was then pulled back in the trachea and passed to the contro-lateral main bronchus. BALF collection was performed again in the same way as for the opposite lung.

The following information was recorded:

- For each horse: The nose in which the tube was introduced and the lung where it was positioned during the first 'blind' BAL.
- For each BAL: the quantity of fluid injected and retrieved.

Each BALF sample (two per horse) was divided into 4 aliquot in EDTA tubes:
- Three tubes were submitted on site to the central Laboratory of Nantes National Vet School (further called 'Lab 1') and were prepared by centrifugation and May Grunwald Giemsa (MGG) stain. Aliquot1 was prepared immediately after submission, Aliquot2 after 24 hours conservation at 4 °C, Aliquot3 after 24 hours at room temperature.
- Aliquot4 was sent to Frank Duncombe Laboratory in Caen (France) (further called 'Lab 2') by postal fast service and was treated the day following the collection. The MGG stain was applied to slides prepared after cytocentrifugation (Cytospin, Shandon-France).

In both laboratories, differential cell count was performed with a minimum of 200 cells. Each cell type was expressed as a percentage of total nucleated cells. All results are presented as mean ± s.d. For comparison of the different groups, a Student t test for paired values was performed. The level of statistical significance was set at $P<0.05$.

The comparison was done between BALF cytological results issued respectively from:
- the right and left lung of the same horse, for all aliquots;
- the same sample treated in Lab1: Aliquots 1, 2 and 3;
- the same sample analyzed after 24 hours at ambient temperature in Lab1 (aliquot 2) and Lab2 (aliquot4).

Results and discussion

In the seven horses, via either right or left ventral nasal meatus, the blind introduction of the tube always yielded to the right main bronchus. Furthermore, some difficulty was often encountered to put the tube into the main left bronchus even with the endoscopic guidance.

In all aliquots, there was no significant difference between right and left lung BALF results for TNCC and cells percentage (Table 1).

In the results issued from Lab1, there was no significant difference between the cytological profiles of the aliquots issued from the same sample (Table 2). However, there was a significant variation in the neutrophil percentage between the results issued respectively from Lab1, aliquot 3 (after 24 hours at room temperature), and from Lab2, aliquot 4 (after 24 hours with postal

Table 1. Mean ± SD results of cytological analysis of BALF issued respectively from right and left lungs (n=7 horses)[1].

	Lab1 – Aliquot1 (immediate treatment)		Lab1 – Aliquot2		Lab1 – Aliquot3		Lab2 – Aliquot4	
	Left	Right	Left	Right	Left	Right	Left	Right
TNCC[2]	441±170[a]	530±187[a]	446±249[a]	424±149[a]	398±210[a]	443±158[a]	422±244[a]	316±68.0[a]
% Ne	20.3±30.8[a]	33.3±28.9[a]	17.0±19.6[a]	20.1±24.0[a]	21.7±21.6[a]	27.0±24.3[a]	16.9±14.1[a]	20.7±21[a]
% Ly	13.9±8.4[a]	9.3±9.3[a]	12.6±7.4[a]	10.6±7.2[a]	11.0±9.4[a]	10.4±8.9[a]	19.6±15.1[a]	14.6±10.9[a]
% Ma	64.6±27.2[a]	56.6±26.1[a]	68.8±21.4[a]	68.4±20.5[a]	66.1±20.3[a]	61.6±19.7[a]	61.4±14.4[a]	63±20.9[a]
% Mast	1.0±1.1[a]	0.4±0.5[a]	1.4±1.6[a]	0.8±0.9[a]	0.8±1.6[a]	0.4±0.8[a]	0.3±0.5[a]	0.1±0.4[a]
% Eo	0.3±0.7[a]	0.4±0.8[a]	1.4±0.4[a]	0±0.0[a]	0.3±0.5[a]	0.6±0.5[a]	0.3±0.5[a]	0.1±0.4[a]

[1] Values with different superscripts are significantly different at $P<0.05$.
[2] TNCC = Total Nucleated Cell Count.

Table 2. Cytological results issued from the different treatments of the samples. n=14 samples (left and right lungs, 7 horses)[1].

	Lab1 Aliquot1 (immediate)	Lab1 Aliquot2 (24H - 4 °C)	Lab1 Aliquot3 (24H – room T°)	Lab2 Aliquot4 (24H – ambient T°)
TNCC[2]	486±178[a]	435±198[a]	421±180[a]	374±186[a]
% Neutrophils	26.8±28.6[a,b]	18.6±21.2[a,b]	24.4±22.2[a]	18.8±17.3[b]
% Lymphocytes	11.6±8.8[a]	11.6±7.1[a]	10.7±8.8[a]	17.1±12.9[a]
% Macrophages	60.6±26.0[a]	68.6±20.1[a]	63.9±19.4[a]	62.2±17.2[a]
% Mast Cells	0.7±0.9[a]	1.1±1.3[a]	0.6±1.2[a]	0.2±0.4[a]
% Eosinophils	0.4±0.7[a]	0.07±0.27[a]	0.4±0.5[a]	0.2±0.4[a]

[1] Values are mean ± s.d. Values with different superscripts are significantly different at $P<0.05$.
[2] TNCC = Total Nucleated Cell Count.

transmission, at ambient temperature – Table 2). This is in accordance with a previous study (Pickles *et al.*, 2002b) in which significant differences had been found between macrophages, lymphocytes, eosinophils and mast cells percentages on cytocentrifuged compared to smear preparations. The authors also showed that smear preparations were reliable for the cytological diagnosis of equine neutrophilic pulmonary disease (Pickles *et al.*, 2002b). Differences in preparation and staining, but also manipulations during postal shipment may explain these differences.

IAD is defined as BALF nuclear cell content with more than 10% neutrophils (Couetil *et al.*, 2007). When this diagnosis criteria is applied to BALF obtained from the right lung (where the tube was blindly introduced in all cases) 4 horses (57%) had evidence of IAD whatever the conservation, treatment and analysis of the aliquot. Two horses had evidence of IAD for 3 of the 4 aliquots. Neutrophil percentage was ≤10% for aliquot 2 treated in Lab1 after 24H of conservation at 4 °C. For the last horse, there was evidence of IAD according to aliquots 1 and 3 but not for aliquots 2 and 4 (Table 3). These results are different from Pickles *et al.* (2002c) study where the time taken for a significant reduction in Total nucleated cell count (TCC) and cell viability of unfixed BALF samples decreased as the storage temperature increased (Pickles *et al.*, 2002c).

Even in the absence of significant statistical difference, great variation in individual neutrophils percentages were observed: one horse had 58% of neutrophils in the right BALF and 3% in the left sample in Lab1, and 16% and 7% respectively in the right and left samples in Lab2. Polynuclear cells are more susceptible than other cells to rapid degeneration, which can in part explain that they are more influenced by condition of submission and preparation of the sample.

This study was conducted with BAL performed at rest on not working horses, without evidence of EIPH. Further studies are needed to evaluate the influence of the sampling site and conditions of conservation on the cellular counts for erythrocytes and haemosiderophages in horses with evidence of EIPH.

Table 3. Individual cytological for aliquots 1, 2, 3 and 4 and for right and left lungs. Bold characters indicate horses with >10% neutrophils (IAD).

Horse	Aliquot1		Aliquot2		Aliquot3		Aliquot4	
	Right	Left	Right	Left	Right	Left	Right	Left
1	**83%**	**89%**	**68%**	**60%**	**80%**	**60%**	**68%**	**47%**
2	**15%**	3%	8%	9%	**11%**	8%	8%	5%
3	**58%**	3%	**12%**	**19%**	**29%**	**18%**	**16%**	7%
4	**18%**	**19%**	0%	7%	**13%**	8%	**13%**	**12%**
5	**29%**	**12%**	**35%**	5%	**24%**	5%	**12%**	**13%**
6	**12%**	6%	3%	6%	**19%**	9%	**14%**	**15%**
7	**18%**	10%	**15%**	**13%**	**13%**	**44%**	**14%**	**19%**

Conclusion

No statistical difference could be demonstrated between cytological profile of BALF issued from right and left lung of the same horse. However neutrophil percentage was influenced by technique of preparation and/or conditions of shipment to the laboratory. Neutrophils are the principal group of cells to define IAD. Therefore care should be taken when interpreting results from different laboratories.

References

Couetil, L.L., Denicola, D.B. (1999) Blood gas, plasma lactate and bronchoalveolar lavage cytology analysis in racehorses with respiratory disease. Equine Veterinary Journal, 30, 77-82.

Couetil, L.L., Hoffman, A.M., Hodgson, J., Buechner-Maxwell, V., Viel, L., Wood, J.L., Lavoie, J.P. (2007) Inflammatory airway disease of horses. Journal of veterinary Internal Medicine, 21, 356-361.

Courouće-Malblanc, A., Pronost, S., Fortier, G., Corde, R., Rossignol, F. (2002) Physiological measurements and upper and lower respiratory tract evaluation in French Standardbred Trotters during a standardized exercise test on the treadmill. Equine Exercise Physiology 6, Equine Vet J. Suppl., 402-407.

Fogarty, U. (1990) Evaluation of a bronchoalveolar lavage technique. Equine vet J. 22(10): 174-176.

Mansmann, R.A., King, C. (1998) How to Perform a Bronchoalveolar Lavage in Practice. Proceeding AAEP; vol44: 186-188.

Pickles, K., Pirie, R.S., Rhind, S., Dixon, P.M., McGorum, B.C. (2002) Cytological analysis of equine bronchoalveolar lavage fluid. Part 1: Comparison of sequential and pooled aliquots. Equine Veterinary Journal 34 (3), pp. 288-291

Pickles, K., Pirie, R.S., Rhind, S., Dixon, P.M., McGorum, B.C. (2002) Cytological analysis of equine bronchoalveolar lavage fluid. Part 2: Comparison of smear and cytocentrifuged preparations. Equine Veterinary Journal 34 (3), 292-296.

Pickles, K., Pirie, R.S., Rhind, S., Dixon, P.M., McGorum, B.C. (2002) Cytological analysis of equine bronchoalveolar lavage fluid. Part 3: The effect of time, temperature and fixatives. Equine Veterinary Journal 34 (3), 297-301

Sweeney, C.R., Rossier, Y., Ziemer, E.L., *et al.* (1992) Effects of lung site and fluid volume on results of broncho-alveolar lavage fluid analysis in horses. Am J Vet Res 53(8): 1376-1379.

Waldridge, B.M., Welles, E.G. (2006) How to Perform a Bronchoalveolar Lavage Using a Three meter Gastroscope. Proceeding AAEP 52: 102-106.

Performance evaluation and management of race and sport horses before, during and after the competitive season

Elizabeth Davidson
University of Pennsylvania, New Bolton Center, 382 W. Street Rd., Kenneth Square, Philadelphia PA 19348, USA

What is performance?

The horse is an amazing athlete which is able to run, turn, and jump over a variety of surfaces while bearing the weight of a rider or driver. When evaluating a horse for performance, considerations must be made for the type and the demands of the competition. Successful racehorses must outperform their fellow competitors by crossing the finish line first. Non-racing performance horse (sport horse) athletic ability is more difficult to define. Its performance is often subjectively judged and compared to the other competitors. It may be the elegance of a particular movement or the sheer jumping ability. Regardless of the type of competition, for the horse to perform adequately, its athletic ability is dependant on coordination movements and complex relations of many body systems.

Performance testing

From time to time, evaluation of the horse's performance is needed. Ideally, performance testing is performed while the horse is actually training or competing. Obvious practical limitations exist with this type of testing; therefore, in most instances athletic function is assessed in different setting and inference to competition performance is based on those findings. Preferably, the testing is completed under conditions that are identical or similar to that of the competition, for example, evaluation of the horse where the ground surface and the horse's gaits, and speeds are similar to those during its actual competition (e.g. field testing). Testing under these conditions also takes the rider or driver into consideration. The disadvantage with this type of testing is that conditions may change on a daily basis, e.g. softer ground after a hard rain. An alternative method of testing is under controlled and repeatable conditions such as with treadmill evaluation. One considerable advantage of a treadmill testing is the accessibility of more equipment for assessing physiological parameters. However, horses do not run on treadmills during competitions. For the most part, field testing has the advantage of specificity while treadmill tests have the advantage of standardization.

Field testing

The biggest advantage of field testing is its similarity to conditions that are used in competition. Another obvious advantage is that it is commonly performed where the horse is stabled for training or competition which is a preferred convenience for the horse owners, trainers and riders. Field testing also allows the evaluation of the horse in the company of other horses, over different gradients and obstacles; however, these factors can also be disadvantages because they can contribute to the difficulties of standardized field exercise tests. Evaluation of gait (soundness or lameness assessment) is best performed in the field since the treadmill locomotion is quite different to that in 'real life'. This is particularly true for non-racing performance horses in which specific movements are required. For example the dressage piaffe, can not be adequately replicated on the treadmill.

The major disadvantage of field testing is the limitation to the number of variables that can be assessed. In the past, field testing was limited to simple tests such as measuring exercising heart rate while most other more sophisticated testing was performed immediately before or immediately after exercise. Recent advancements in technology have greatly improved the ability to assess cardiac and upper respiratory function in the field. Currently, over-ground telemetric equipment is commercially available and is increasingly utilized. The telemetric ECG system Televet 100® uses Bluetooth® technology and can record heart rhythm from a distance of approximately 100 meters. The DRS® (Dynamic Respiratory Scope) system utilizes a backpack for electronics and lavage system which is secured to the rider's back, saddle pad or harness and the flexible endoscope is secured in position via a specialized bridle. This system also includes a handheld viewer for direct visualization of the upper airway. Both telemetric systems utilize a SD card to record and download data to a laptop computer or a handheld computerized device. While testing portability continues to improve, there still remain limitations.

Treadmill testing

High-speed treadmill (HSTM) evaluation has the advantage of standardizing testing variables. Speeds, duration, and slope of the treadmill can be controlled and exercise protocols are repeatable. Although what is 'standard HSTM testing' is different among various veterinary institutions, the overall concept is similar. Typical testing first involves familiarization; the horse is acclimated to the treadmill and associated equipment. The actual exercise test consists of a warm up phase of walking, trotting and moderate canter (or trotting/pacing for Standardbred racehorses) followed by a high-speed test at as fast a speed as the individual horse is capable of sustaining for 1600 to 2400 meters. The exact intensity of the high-speed test is dictated by the temperament, fitness, and ability of an individual horse but in most maximal speeds will approach 12 to 14 m/s. For some horses, the uphill exercise may be appropriate; this is especially true for horses used in competitions that include jumping (i.e. steeple chasing, eventing). Treadmill belts are usually rubber which provides an even, consistent and stable surface. However, the belt is firmer than most other exercising ground surfaces and repetitive impact while exercising on the treadmill can lead to injury. Minimizing the training time and maximizing the exercise effort (running on a sloped treadmill) can reduce the possibility of injury.

Another advantage of treadmill evaluation is the multitude of tests that can be performed on what is, in effect, a stationary horse. The most common instrumentation includes telemetric ECG recording system, catheterization of a systemic artery (e.g. transverse facial artery) for serial blood gas analysis, a means of measuring core body temperature, and placement of an endoscopy to visualize the upper airway. Facemasks and indwelling catheters for airway pressures can be utilized to assess airflow mechanics; however, are usually reserved for research purposes.

Disadvantages of treadmill testing are that the horse is exercised without a rider and exercising on a rubber belt in a straight ward motion (no turning or jumping). The apparatus does require some acclimation training and not all horses are amenable to treadmill exercise. In addition, treadmill gaits are different to those on ground surfaces and therefore limit effective assessment of the musculoskeletal system.

Factors limiting performance

Peak performance requires all body systems to function at or close to their maximum capacity. For healthy horses, performance-limiting factor(s) depends on the type of exercise. In racehorses, running at top speed is limited by oxygen transport. Any reduction, for example decrease in laryngeal diameter secondary to recurrent laryngeal neuropathy, will diminish the performance capacity of the respiratory system which will in turn affect the rest of the body systems. However if the performance does not require peak effort, impairments in physiological functions may be tolerable. For example a dressage horse with recurrent laryngeal neuropathy may be able to perform (although the associated abnormal respiratory noise may detract from its performance). An understanding of what is likely to limit performance for each breed and use of horse is important not only in understanding the physiology of that form of exercise, but also in determining the likely causes of poor performance in horses with clinical disease.

In the client owned horse, performance testing is usually performed to investigate for factors which are limiting performance e.g. testing decline in performance or poor performance. The fewer the possible factors which contribute to the performance (or lack there of), the more likely the testing will provide useful information. For example, in a racehorse that is making a loud consistent abnormal respiratory noise during exercise, exercising endoscopy is very likely to reveal a definitive answer.

Poor performance testing

When one or more systems 'break down' and the horse is no longer able to perform up to his potential, testing is focused on the reasons for diminished ability. In some cases, the cause for the poor performance is quite obvious. For example, the horse with a severe musculoskeletal injury will be severely lame. However, in many instances, the horse has a subtle or gradual decline in performance and has few or no distinct abnormal clinical findings. Common complaints from their riders/trainers/owners may include trailing off at the end of competition, long recovery, or just not right.

Taking into account the number and complexity of mechanisms involved in a good performer, investigation of poor performance or loss of performance can be a real challenge. This is when real detective work begins. It starts with obtaining a clear and accurate history followed by a thorough physical examination. It may also involve numerous diagnostics, the expertise of multiple clinicians, and a good laboratory for cytological and hematological analysis.

Since musculoskeletal injury is the most common cause for loss of performance, poor performance evaluation should include a thorough musculoskeletal examination. Overt lameness is easily recognized and an accepted cause for poor performance, but mild or subtle lameness is often overlooked as a potential cause of decreased performance. A traditional field lameness examination is preferred over treadmill testing; treadmill exercise confuses and masks all but the most severe lameness. Depending on the nature of the gait disorder, specific field exercises (jumping, evaluation under tack, etc.) may also be necessary. As with any thorough lameness examination, perineural analgesia techniques are also recommended to pinpoint the authentic source of pain. Bear in mind that some good performers succeed despite musculoskeletal pain, e.g. the elite show jumper with chronic foot pain that limps in the parking lot but runs and jumps fault free. In any instance, identification of musculoskeletal pain is important but equally important is its impact on the performance.

Recent advancements in technology combined with the vast collective knowledge of veterinary diagnosticians have secured the use of imaging in performance evaluations. Radiography and ultrasonography are routinely used not only for the evaluation of poor performance but also the evaluation of a good performer (e.g. prepurchase examination). Nuclear scintigraphy remains the gold standard for early recognition of a 'stress fracture' before catastrophic injury. Identification of these and other stress related bone injuries is critical in the poor performer since affected horses often have subtle, inconsistent, or multiple limb lameness. CT and MRI are increasingly more available to the equine diagnostician and are especially useful for foot and subchondral diseases.

The prevalence of respiratory disease in all types of competition horses is high and in many cases airway disorders only occur during exercise. Detection of disease is complicated by the absence of clinical signs such as cough and/or nasal discharge and the inability to predict exercising upper airway function based on resting endoscopic findings. Exercising abnormal respiratory noise is a common clinical clue associated with upper airway obstruction; however, as many as 30% of horses with intermittent dorsal displacement of the soft palate do not make a noise. Therefore exercising videoendoscopy is particularly useful and widely used. Numerous treadmill studies have documented the merit of dynamic upper airway endoscopy. Over-ground endoscopy is relatively new; however, early reports regarding is usefulness are promising and it may be particular valuable for assessment of conditions not reproducible during treadmill exercise. Exercising endoscopy has facilitated the diagnosis of a sundry of performance limiting upper airway obstructions. In the show horse, upper airway obstruction may be tolerated despite the presence of noise. Abnormal respiratory noise or exercise intolerance can also be exacerbated by head and neck flexion, a position required or desired for certain disciplines, movements, and gaits of show horses. Lower airway inflammation/disease, another important cause of reduced athletic ability, can be ascertained with lung function testing such as forced oscillometry and/or bronchoalveolar (BAL) cytology. Subclinical lung disease is common in all types of performance horses and can be particularly challenging to diagnosis.

The incidence of cardiac murmurs in performance horses is also high, with mitral and tricuspid valvular regurgitation the most common, although most murmurs are of minimal consequence to performance. Arrhythmias are also common and some dysrhythmias such as atrial fibrillation have been associated with poor performance due to decreased cardiac output. Telemetric exercising ECG assessment either over ground or during treadmill exercise is relatively easy to perform and usually diagnostic. Post-exercise stress echocardiography performed immediately after peak exercise can be a useful tool for assessment of myocardial function.

Management

Good management practices for the performance horse begin with a solid training program. When preparing for competition, the horse should regularly train for the specific tasks that are required in the competition. For example, a horse trained with long slow intensity exercise will be poorly trained for short fast sprints. Training activities should be introduced and then repeated at an intensity that will induce the physiological changes needed for optimal performance. These repetitive exercises induce a multitude of physiological and anatomical adaptations that are sufficient to counteract the stresses they will sustain during the competition. For example, in young Thoroughbred racehorses in race training, cyclical stress placed the dorsal third metacarpi will result in dorsomedial thickening of the cortical on bone. This phenomenon of adaptation /remodeling is common to many body compositions and is vital for the horse to overcome the strains of peak exercise.

When these adaptive processes fail, the body is unable to counteract the stresses of competition resulting in fatigue or failure. This failure may be due to poor or maladaptive changes due to improper training. Using the same young Thoroughbred in race training as an example, periostitis, 'bucked shins', is a maladaptive change in the dorsal metacarpi in which the bony remodeling process was unable to keep up with the repetitive high-cyclic strains resulting in poorly adapted periosteal new bone. Left unrecognized and compounded with increases in bony stress, this poorly adapted cortex may succumb to stress fracture.

Management practices of the poor performer should be focused on the authentic reason for the decline in athletic ability. Since it is often multifactorial, comprehensive performance testing is also recommended. Performance following prosthetic laryngoplasty may be less than expected if accompanying lower airway inflammation is not recognized and treated. However, whole body or 'best guess' treatments should be used with caution since they may prolong disease identification or worsen the injury. Clearly early and accurate recognition of the causes of declined performance followed by appropriate management practices is vital to the welfare and safety of the performance horse.

References

Birks, E.K., Durando, M.M., Marin, B.B. (2004) Clinical exercise testing: evaluation of the poor performing athlete. In: Hinchcliff, K.W., Kaneps, A.J., Goer, R.J. (eds.), Equine Sports Medicine and Surgery. Saunders, pp 9-18.

Desmaizieres, L.-M., Serraud, N., Plainfosse, B. *et al.* (2009) Dynamic respiratory endoscopy without treadmill in 68 performance Standardbred, Thoroughbred and saddle horses under natural training conditions. Eq Vet J 41, 347-352.

Evans, D.L. (2008) Exercise testing in the field. In: Hinchcliff, K.W., Geor, R.J., Kaneps, A.J. (eds.), Equine Exercise Physiology. Saunders, pp 12-27.

Martin, B.B., Reef, V.B., Parente, E.J. *et al.* (2000) Causes of poor performance of horses during racing, training, or showing: 348 cases (1992-1996). J Am Vet Assoc 216, 554-558.

Morris, E.A., Seeherman, H.J. (1990) Evaluation of upper respiratory tract function during strenuous exercise in racehorses. J Am Vet Assoc 196, 431-438.

Pollock, P.J., Reardon, R.J.M., Parkin, T.D.H. *et al.* (2009) Dynamic respiratory endoscopy in 67 Thoroughbred racehorses training under normal ridden exercise conditions. Eq Vet J 41, 354-360.

Clinical significance of side bones in Cold-Blooded Trotters

Ulf Hedenström[1] and Ove Wattle[2]
[1]National Equine Centre for Trotting, Wången, Alsen, Sweden
[2]Section for Large Animal Medicine and Surgery, Department of Clinical Sciences, Swedish University of Agricultural Sciences, Uppsala, Sweden

Take-home message

There was no clinical significance of side bones regarding racing performance in Cold-Blooded Trotters. The radiograph grading system suggested by Ruohoniemi *et al.* (1993) may be improved using more steady skeletal structures as reference points.

Introduction

The Cold-Blooded Trotter is a slightly heavier breed than the Standardbred Trotter, with high performing potential, a long career, and the capacity to be trained and raced at high speed (>10 m/s) on different, but often hard, surfaces.

Historically, ossification of the collateral cartilages of the third phalanx (so-called side bones, SB) has been classified as a malady and in some breeds, such as the Cold-Blooded Trotter, sires with high grades of SB have been excluded from breeding. Regardless of grade, it is still unclear whether SB is a disease or whether it just reflects normal physiological variation. Irrespective of etiology, it is also unclear whether SB influences a horse's performance.

A variety of grading systems have been used over the years. Since the mid-1980s, the radiograph grading system suggested by Ruohoniemi *et al.* (1993) has been used when evaluating Cold-Blooded Trotters. Clinically, when comparing radiographs taken on different occasions from the same horse, the borders of the navicular bone have proven to be an uncertain point of reference. Thus, variations in technique when taking radiographs, in hoof form, and in the amount of limb loading can affect the position of the navicular bone within the hoof capsule.

The aim of the present study was to determine whether SB has any influence on the racing performance of Cold-Blooded Trotters. Furthermore, we wanted to evaluate a radiological grading system that reflects the grade of SB in a more repeatable, and thereby more clinically relevant, way. Our hypothesis was that SB does not affect the performance of Cold-Blooded Trotters.

Material and methods

Two hundred and twenty-nine Swedish Cold-Blooded Trotters, 133 male and 96 female, born between 1971 and 2001 were included in this study. Dorso-palmar radiographs of front hooves were taken in connection with inclusion of Cold-Blooded Trotters through open invitations to horse owners living in the vicinity of race tracks and equine clinics. Sixty-three of the horses (corresponding to 252 cartilages) were also re-examined after a minimum of four years (mean 9 years, median 10). All radiographs were blinded and evaluated regarding SB using the 0-5 point scale of Ruohoniemi and co-workers (1993) (RG) as well as on a scale from 0 to 3 (NS), Figure 1. To forgive the naturally occurring variability in shape of the distal phalanx, our grade 1 starts at the distal border of the second phalanx (PII) and ends at our grade 2. The demarcation for ossification of grade 2 is between the proximal border of the distal interphalangeal joint and the mid-level of PII.

Grading according to Ruohoniemi:
- Grade 0: No ossification, inclination sagitally.
- Grade 1: Ossification at the base of the cartilage.
- Grade 2: Proximal to grade 1 but not above the level of the central part of the fovea articularis of the second phalanx.
- Grade 3: To the level of proximal border of the navicular bone (dotted line).
- Grade 4: Proximal to the navicular bone but not above the distal half of P2.
- Grade 5: Ossification above the distal half of P2.

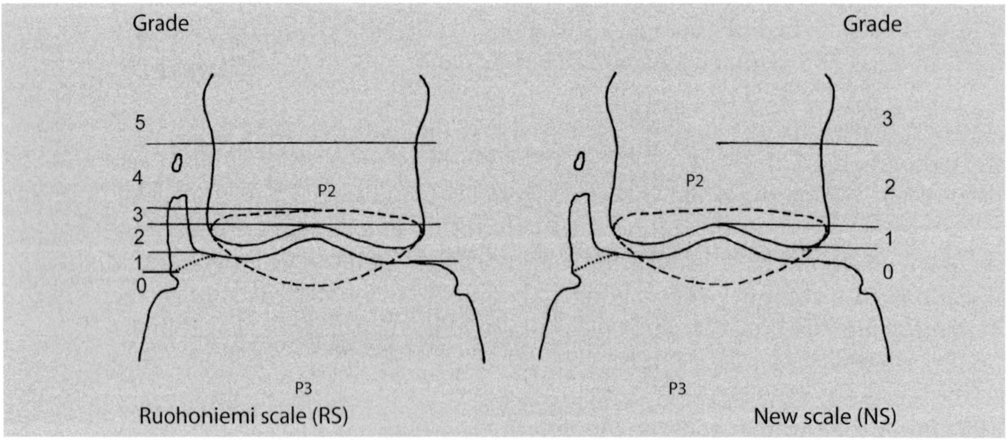

Figure 1. Grading of ossification. The left panel illustrates moderate ossification with separate centre of ossification. The dotted line illustrates the navicular bone. P2 and P3 refer to the second and third phalanx.

New grading scale:

- Grade 0: SB not proximal to distal P2.
- Grade 1: Ossification proximal to distal P2 but not above the level of the central part of the fovea articularis of the second phalanx.
- Grade 2: Proximal to grade 1 but not above the distal half of P2.
- Grade 3: Ossification above the distal half of P2.

Of the 4 hoof cartilages evaluated per horse, the one with the highest degree of ossification counted as the score for the horse. Average best linear unbiased prediction (BLUP) index and reliable sports data were collected from the databases of the Swedish and Norwegian trotting associations. Data on the relationship between money gained, number of starts, and time record on the one hand and grade of SB on the other were analyzed using general linear models. The models also included the sex of the horse. *P*-values <0.05 were considered significant.

Results

Using the Ruohoniemi grading system and our new grading system, ossification of the collateral cartilages was found in 65% and 21% of the horses, respectively. Depending on the position of the navicular bone, 3 horses had a lower grade of SB when the radiographs taken at the re-examination were evaluated with RS while there was no reduction in the grade of SB when using the NS. High-grade ossification, i.e. grade 4 or 5 with RS and grade 2 or 3 with NS, was found in 4% of the horses. Of the 229 horses included, 170 (74%) had competed. The incidence of SB was not significantly different between the group of horses that had started and those that had not competed at all. Of the 63 horses that were re-examined, 71% had competed. The incidence of SB was 38% in this population and also in the 13 of the re-examined horses that had not competed. For horses that were older than 2 years at the time of the first radiographic examination, there was no significant increase in amount of ossification between the two examinations. Mean BLUP index of the original population, as well as for horses that had competed and horses that never started, was 97. Average money gained, number of starts, and time record as of August 2009 was SEK 108,000, 35 races, and 1.32 min/km (11 m/s), respectively. Money gained, number of starts, and record time were not significantly associated with the presence of SB.

Conclusion

The incidence of SB corresponded to earlier reports regarding breed and sex. Our new grading system was found to be more forgiving regarding variations in technique, hoof form, and loading between the two examinations but gave equally relevant clinical information. We propose that a system that excludes the navicular bone as reference for ossification and that accepts variability in the shape of the distal phalanx is more clinically relevant. Moreover, for horses older than 2 years at the time of the first radiographs, we could not detect any significant increase in the grade of ossification between the two sets of radiographs. We could not find any significant effect of side bones on the performance of the Cold-Blooded Trotter. Considering the fact that the horses had trained, and that most of them had also competed frequently during the years between the two examinations, it is reasonable to conclude that the workload does not affect the incidence of SB in Cold-Blooded Trotters.

References

Arnason, T., (1999). Genetic evaluation of Swedish standard-bred trotters for racing performance traits and racing status. J. Anim. Breed. Genet. 116, 387-398.

Ruohoniemi, M., Tulamo, R.M., Hackzell, M. (1993). Radiographic evaluation of ossification of the collateral cartilages of third phalanx in Finnhorses. Equine vet. J. 25(5): 453-455.

Therapeutic applications of stem cells obtained from peripheral blood in tendons, ligaments and skin injuries

Valentina Martini, Patrizia Palomba, Marco Ranalli, Graziella Zohar, Carlotta Gabbiani, Marco Polettini and Alessandra Gambacurta
[1]Dept. of Sperimental Medicine and Sciences, Faculty of Medicine and Surgery, University of Roma 'Tor Vergata', Italy

Take home message

A new method to obtain and use stem cells directly from mammal's peripheral blood cells (Patent N. IT RM 2006A000498) in a quick and relatively easy way is presented.

Introduction

The term 'stem cells' designates cells which have the capability of self-renewal and the capability to form at least one and often a number of specialized cell types due to their asymmetrical division capability. The term 'pluripotent' indicates stem cells, which can differentiate into all possible cell types of the body.

Stem cells can be isolated from different tissues of adult individuals. Such stem cells are referred to as 'multipotent adult stem cells'. In the body they play a role in tissue regeneration and homeostasis. The actual problems relating to the obtaining and use of adult stem cells however lie in the rarity of these cells. Thus, in the bone marrow, stem cells are present only in the ratio of 1:10,000, in the peripheral blood of 1:250,000 and in the liver in the ratio of 1:100,000. At the moment, obtaining such stem cells and the generation of large quantities, as required for clinical therapy, is therefore very expensive and stressful for the patient.

In veterinary medicine the bone marrow is currently the main source of equine MSCs but, bone marrow derived autologous MSCs require time consuming, in vitro propagation prior to transplantation and a decreased yield of stem cells from the bone marrow with increasing age makes the technique age-dependent which is paradoxical to the fact that many clinical cases are aged individuals.

There are no peer-reviewed reports of equine adipose tissue derived stem cells although commercial marketing of so-called equine adipose tissue derived stem cell therapy is done. There appears to be no published studies on equine cord blood or mesenchymal stem cells, although commercial storage of equine cord blood for possible future autologous stem cell transplantations is available. Isolation of pluripotent stem cells from equine blood provides a non-invasive source of stem cells with potentially superior cellular characteristics to other equine stem cells with regard to immune tolerance, proliferative potential and differentiation potency. Our study reports a new method to obtain and expand pluripotent stem cells from the blood and their use in several pathologies. These cells, as shown by cytofluorimetric analysis, express all the typical markers characterizing pluripotent stem cells, such as CD90, CD117, CD105, Sox2, Oct3/4 and Nanog.

Noticeable, preliminary *in vitro* experiments show that the same method of purification and expansion can be used for human blood too, allowing a great enrichment of mesenchymal stem cells in the sample. In vivo our cells have demonstrated the ability to regenerate several different tissues. In this work we report how this cells can be used in injuries of tendons (superficial and deep digital flexor tendons), ligaments (collateral ligament of distal interphalangeal joint, suspensory ligament, lig. sesamoideum rectum, distal oblique sesamoidean ligament) and skin (2th-3th degree burns, antibiotic resistant infections).

Material and methods

Stem cells isolation and cultivation

Each blood sample of about 5-7 ml was taken from the lower limbs and immediately put into test tubes containing heparin or EDTA as anticoagulant to prevent clotting. Immediately after collection, samples were stored on ice.

Preparation of Peripheral Blood Stem Cells was achieved as follows. Blood samples were diluted 1:3 in NH_4Cl (1M), centrifuged at 3.023 g and washed several times with PBS (Dulbecco A, OXOID Limited Basingstoke Hampshire, England) to remove any red cells contamination. After erythrocytes removal the pellet was dissolved in 5ml of PBS. The nucleated cells were incubated for at least 72 hours at 37 °C with MCSF.

Cytofluorimetric analyses

After the expansion cells were analyzed for number and phenotype by FACSARIAII cytofluorometric analysis and eventually incubated, again, for 24 hours with MCFS 45 nM before sorting. For their immuno-phenotyping characterization cells were centrifuged and the pellet dissolved in 5ml of PBS (Dulbecco A, OXOID Limited Basingstoke Hampshire, England). 200 μL were taken for each analyses and were incubated at room temperature for 30 minutes with saturating amounts of human antibodies alone or in combination CD90-PE (BD Biosciences, San Jose, USA), CD117-APC (BD Biosciences, San Jose, USA), CD34-PerCp (BD Biosciences, San Jose, USA), CD 105-FITC (BD Biosciences, San Jose, USA) and CD14-PE (Biolegend). After acquisition samples were filtered

(50 μ Syringe Filcons Sterile BD Biosciences, San Jose, USA). Cells were analyzed by flow cytometric analysis using a FACSAriaII flow cytometer equipped with blue, red and violet lasers and DIVA software (BD Biosciences, San Jose, USA) with a minimum of 10,000 events acquired. After ultrasound localization of the SDFT, cells were sorted to obtain the necessary cells number for the local treatment or centrifuged and re-suspended in PBS and gentamicine 5uM for intravenous treatments.

Local and ntravenous therapy

The cells were inoculated directly in the site of the tendon, ligament or skin lesion; in cases where the cells could not be inserted precisely in the lesions the following method was used:

- for lesions to collateral ligaments the injection was made between the second and third phalanx.

Cells were used intravenously one or more times.

Variables that influenced the quantity of cells administered are: seriousness of the pathology, age and general conditions of patient, if acute or chronic.

Cases treated

230 spontaneous tendon and ligament injuries: 50% superficial digital flexor tendon, 10% superficial digital flexor tendon, 25% suspensory ligament, 10% collateral ligament of the distal interphalangeal joint, 5% others.

Typology of evaluated horses: 50% jumping horses, 10% eventing horses, 10% dressage horses, 10% quarter horses, 10% thoroughbred horses, 10% others. 50% geldings, 5% male, 45% female from 2 to 25 years. Follow-up examinations were performed at approximately 40, 70 and 120 days for clinical and ultrasonic healing and return to soundness. In this work we treated 25 horses with spontaneous skin wounds resistant to conventional therapies (14 geldings, 1 male, 10 female from 4 to 22 years). All the patients were treated with blood stem cells by intravenous and local administration.

Results

In vitro

We present the phenotypic analyses after in vitro expansion by FACSAriaII cytofluorimetric analysis on sorted stem cells derived from peripheral blood. We identify in vitro at least three subpopulations

- A typical hematopoietic stem cell population, positive for CD90, CD117 and CD34
- A 'mesenchymal stem cell like' population, showing CD105, CD50 expression
- A 'pluripotent-like stem cells' population, expressing the intracellular transcription factors Sox2, Oct3/4 and Nanog.

These factors have been shown to be strongly involved in the maintenance of the undifferentiated state of pluripotent cells. In addition to the above mentioned markers we also found some positivity for CXCR4, CD29, CD49e and CD49b molecules.

In vivo

The ultrasound analysis demonstrate that tendon's and ligament's injuries after 40 days present a good reorganization of the fibres, after about 120 days are almost completely solved. In this work we also consider the return of the horses to full work and soundness and the performances obtained (mainly in steeple-chase, 3 day event and thoroughbred races where relapses are more frequent) as an evaluation factor of this therapy's potency. For skin wounds we achieved the healing in a time from 10 to 120 days, all the changes were recorded taking photographs regularly. The success depended on dimension and chronicity of wound.

Conclusions

Adult stem cells function is to facilitate tissue repair by replacing lost or damaged specialized resident cells. The ability to obtain in less than 72 hours a large number of autologous pluripotent stem cells from an easily accessible and un-invasive source such as peripheral blood, the possibility to use them both by local and/or by systemic way, should make them valuable candidates for a lot of therapeutic protocols, also for degenerative systemic pathologies. Peripheral blood stem cells can be used to treat severe lesions in tendons, ligaments and skin. The ultrasound recording of the evolution of severe tendon's (3rd and 4th degree) and ligament's injuries, supported by sport performances of our patients proved our treatment protocol's effectiveness. Anyway we must always detect and solve lesion's causes (metabolic, environmental, conformation, biomechanics) to prevent relapses. In six years, none of the animal treated so far has shown any side effect such as phenomena of rejection, infection or the onset of teratomi.

Functional electrical stimulation (FES) for use in equine medicine

Sheila J. Schils
Equine Rehabilitation, EquiNew, LLC, United Kingdom

Take Home Message

Functional electrical stimulation (FES) is a distinct class of electrotherapy that replicates the motor neuron response to produce true muscle contractions. Case studies show the applicability of FES to reverse muscle wasting and decrease muscle spasticity.

Introduction

Functional Electrical Stimulation (FES) is a neuromuscular electrical stimulation (NMES) which replicates the motor neuron response to illicit motor and sensory stimulation. FES produces true muscular movement, which makes it distinctly different from other classes of electrotherapy devices, such as transcutaneous electrical nerve stimulators (TENS), interferential, high-voltage pulsed or galvanic (Robinson and Snyder-Mackler, 2008).

FES is the most applicable of the electrotherapy devices for use in veterinary medicine due to the stimulation of both sensory and motor neurons and the ability to activate the superficial and deep muscles of the horse. There is high compliance to the treatments even when deep muscles are stimulated due to the production of muscle contractions that feel 'normal' to the horse (Schils, 2009). Whenever controlled muscular movement would be appropriate for healing or strengthening, FES can be utilized. The purpose of this paper is to review the use of FES as a treatment protocol for equine medicine through the discussion of two case studies.

Materials and methods

FES is a microprocessor-controlled device, which generates an electrical impulse that is transmitted to surface electrodes. When the intensity of the FES reaches a sufficient level, an action potential is produced in the muscle or nerve resulting in a functional muscle reaction. The ability to produce functional movement is what defines the FES system from all other electrical stimulation modalities. For example, the application of FES to the appropriate muscles of the hand can produce a precise gripping action.

Due to the massiveness of the equine muscular system, when compared to the human, the intensity of the signal is of utmost importance or the deeper muscles of the horse will not be affected. However, at a high intensity the signal must closely replicate the electrical charges of the body so that the treatment is as comfortable as it is effective.

The amount of research available on the use of electrotherapy for human rehabilitation is extensive. The American Physical Therapy Association acknowledges the use of electrotherapy to:

- manage pain;
- improve range of motion;
- reduce acute and chronic edema;
- improve motor control;
- improve strength;
- reverse muscle wasting;
- repair tissue (especially slow to heal wounds);
- improve blood and lymphatic flow (Alon *et al.*, 2005).

The FES system can be used with surface electrodes on groups of muscles and the associated tendons, individual muscles, or 'trigger points' to elicit sensory or motor responses. Joint movement can be produced when stronger muscle contractions are obtained. Electrodes are placed in a pad that is administered to the treatment site, or self-stick electrodes can be used on any part of the body. Avoidance of the brainstem, carotid artery, metal implants and directly over the heart are the main contraindications for horses. The minimum voltage applied is 0.2 volts, and 20 volts is the typical maximum voltage used to produce muscle contractions. The FES system can also be attached to acupuncture needles for use with electroacupuncture.

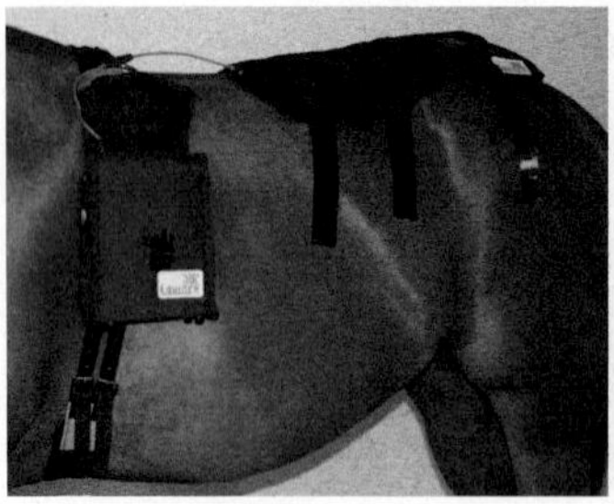
Pad placement on the back

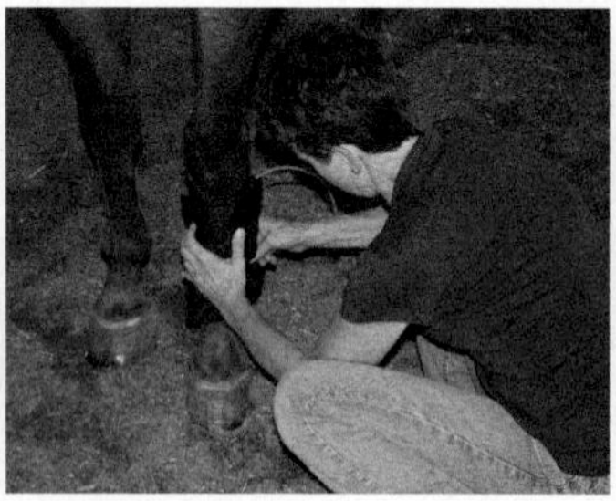
Pad placement on the leg

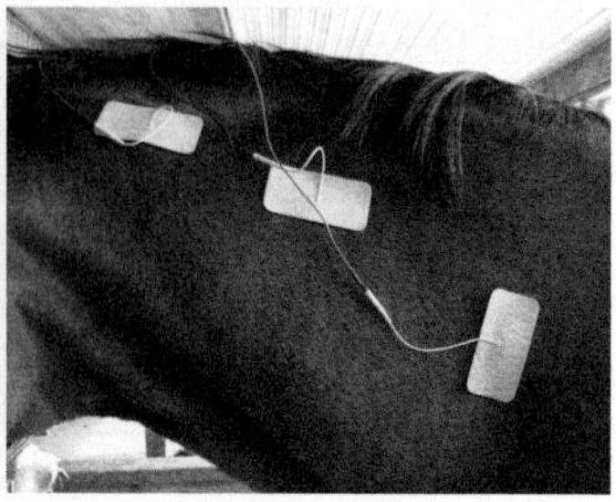
Self-stick electrodes

Examples the use of FES in equine medicine is outlined in the following case studies. These cases were selected because they were treated exclusively with the FES modality and have documentation of the treatment progress. The case studies illustrate two benefits of FES: reduction of muscle atrophy, and decrease of muscle spasticity.

Case Study 1. Reduction of muscle atrophy

Reduction of muscle atrophy in spinal-cord injury patients was one of the original uses of FES in the 1980s. The denervated muscle of para- and quadriplegics was stimulated utilizing FES to produce a cycling movement of the legs that resulted in the reduction of muscle wasting. Since that time, many studies have acknowledged the use of FES to reduce muscle atrophy in humans. Research has shown the specific effect of FES treatments on muscle development through the analysis of muscle biopsies. In this study, human subjects were selected who displayed severe myofiber atrophy. With the use of FES stimulation, the muscle biopsies showed decreased muscle atrophy initially, with almost complete reversal if the treatment was continued (Kern *et al.*, 2005). In another study, the quadriceps of spinal-cord injury patients were stimulated utilizing FES. The maximal electrically stimulated torque of the quadriceps increased fivefold during one year of training with FES used 5 days a week (Duffell *et al.*, 2008). In humans, FES has been shown to be safe in reducing atrophy and improving muscle strength in even the most fragile muscle tissue, denervated muscle (Carraro *et al.*, 2005).

The first case study was an ulna fracture that was surgically repaired with a plate. During recovery, a pronounced atrophy of the triceps developed. FES was utilized on the triceps as well as on the top line from T13-L4. The pictures document the change in the musculature after 9 treatments on the shoulder.

Case Study 2. Decrease of muscle spasticity

The use of FES to reduce spasticity has been reported in the literature. FES was shown to successfully decrease muscle spasticity related to multiple sclerosis in humans (Krause *et al.*, 2007). In addition, FES was utilized for treatment of long-term spasticity in hemiplegic patients which resulted in reduction of spasticity, as well as an improvement in strength (Stefanovska *et al.*, 1989). Stiffness associated with spastic muscle in spinal-cord injury patients was decreased up to 53% with the conclusion that FES helped reduce abnormal joint stiffness (Mirbagheri *et al.*, 2002).

The second case study documents the use of FES on a 'kissing spine' diagnosis. On 11/13/02 the mare was presented as Grade 4/5 hind limb lameness. At the walk in hand, the mare drug both hind toes and was uncoordinated when turning in small circles. She previously had a successful career as a grand prix

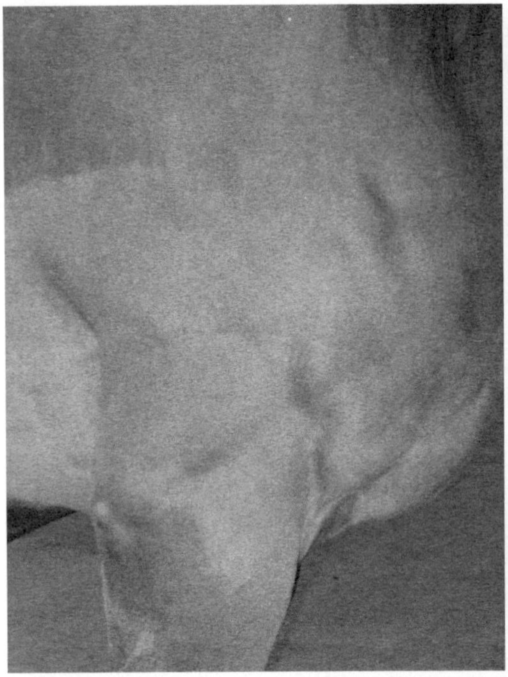

Pre Treatment

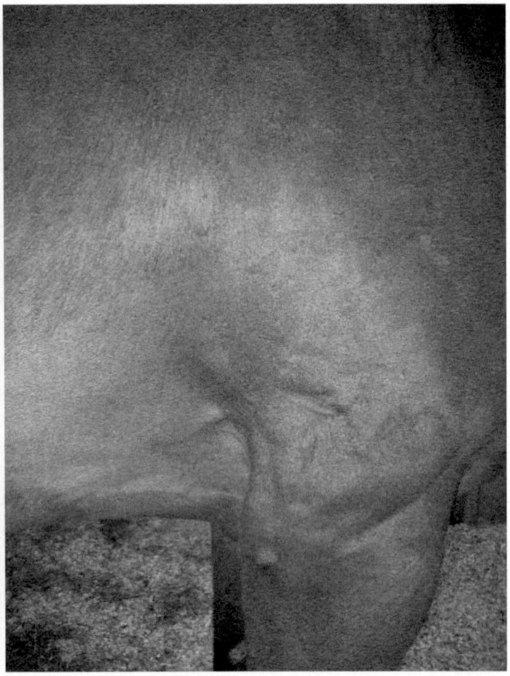

4 FES Treatments

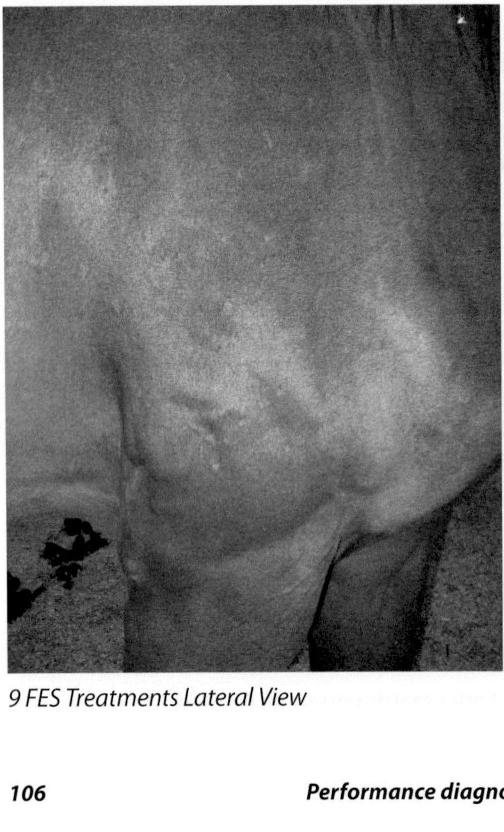

9 FES Treatments Lateral View

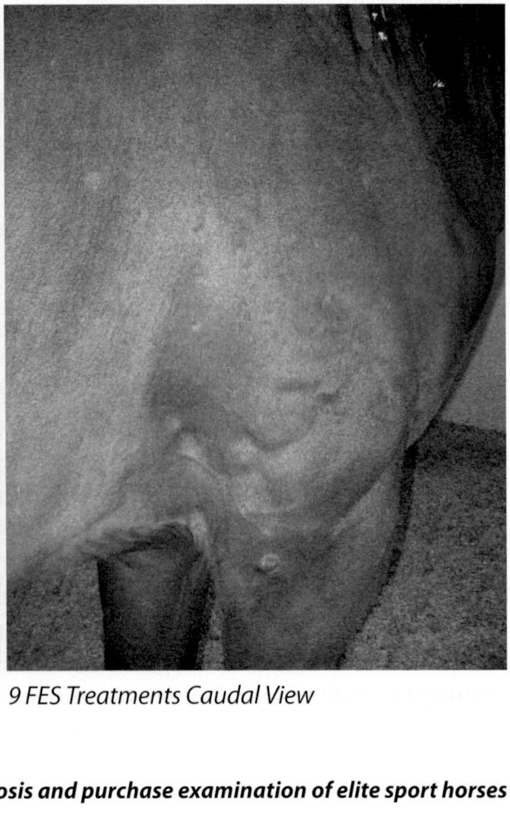

9 FES Treatments Caudal View

jumper. No specific injury was noted, just a progressive decline in performance over the preceding year.

The past history of this case study included 8/7/01 spinal x-rays confirming kissing spine in the posterior thoracic vertebrae. Spinal injections were given at the time of the x-rays. In subsequent months, chiropractic and acupuncture treatments were given. No improvement in performance was noted with any of these treatments.

On 11/13/02 FES treatments were started. Spastic muscles along the top line from T13-L2 were noted as well as spasticity in the gluteal muscle region. The mare was ridden after two FES treatments and the owner noted improvements in the stride length and in the willingness of the mare to move forward.

After 7 treatments, the mare was cantering willingly under saddle and returned to light jumping work of fences under 2'. A total of 17 treatments were given over a period of 5 months. After 5 months of treatments, the mare returned to Grand Prix competition. She was retired 2 years later without any further lameness issues and continues to this day to work as a schoolmaster with no further FES treatments since 2005.

Results and conclusions

Electrotherapy can be an effective modality for treatment of muscular and associated tendon and ligament injuries in horses, however it is not extensively utilized. In part, this may be due to the fact that the devices and treatment protocols must be modified to suit the specific characteristics of the equine musculature. In addition, practitioners need to become familiar with the differences between electrotherapy devices to select the appropriate modality for application. If the electrotherapy treatment is uncomfortable to the horse, or does not activate the targeted musculature, the full benefits of the modality will not be obtained.

Functional electrical stimulation (FES) is a neuromuscular electrical stimulator (NMES) that has been utilized to produce encouraging rehabilitation outcomes in horses. Case studies documenting the use of FES to reverse muscle atrophy and decrease muscle spasticity show the possible outcomes of the use of FES as a treatment modality. An expanding use of FES in the future will provide even further information regarding the usefulness of electrotherapy in equine medicine.

References

Alon, G. *et al.* (2005) Electrotherapeutic Terminology in Physical Therapy; Section on Clinical Electrophysiology. Alexandria, VA: American Physical Therapy Association.

Carraro, U., Rossini, K., Mayr, W., Kern, H. (2005) Muscle fiber regeneration in human permanent lower motoneuron denervation: relevance to safety and effectiveness of FES-training, which induces muscle recovery in SCI subjects. Artif Organs. 29(3): 187-191.

Duffell, L.D., Donaldson, N. Perkins, T.A., Rushton, D.N., Hunt, K.J., Kakebeeke, T.H., Newham, D.J. (2008) Long-term intensive electrically stimulated cycling by spinal cord-injured people: effect on muscle properties and their relation to power output. Muscle Nerve. 38(4): 1304-1311.

Kern, H., Rossini, K., Carraro, U., Mayr, W., Vogelauer, M., Hoellwarth, U., Hofer, C. (2005) Muscle biopsies show that FES of denervated muscles reverses human muscle degeneration from permanent spinal motoneuron lesion. J Rehabil Res Dev. 42(3 Suppl 1): 43-53.

Krause, P., Szecsi, J., Straube, A. (2007) FES cycling reduces spastic muscle tone in a patient with multiple sclerosis. Neurorehabilitation. 22(4): 335-337.

Mirbagheri, M.M., Ladouceur, M., Barbeau, H., Kearney, R.E. (2002) The effects of long-term FES-assisted walking on intrinsic and reflex dynamic stiffness in spastic spinal-cord-injured subjects. IEEE Trans Neural Syst Rehabil Eng. 10(4): 280-289.

Robinson, A.J., Snyder-Mackler, L. (2008) Clinical Electrophysiology: electrotherapy and electrophysiologic testing. 3rd ed. Philadelphia: Lippincott Williams & Wilkins, p. 27-70.

Schils, S.J. (2009) Review of Electrotherapy Devices for Use in Veterinary Medicine. Proceedings 55th Annual AAEP Convention, Las Vegas, p. 68-73.

Stefanovska, A., Vodovnik, L., Gros, N., Rebersek, S., Acimović-Janezic, R.. (1989) FES and spasticity. IEEE Trans Biomed Eng. 36(7): 738-745.

Effects of preliminary transport on the haematological changes of horses after a two-day-trekking event

E. Fazio, P. Medica, E. Giacoppo, R. Pellizzotto, C. Cravana and A. Ferlazzo
Department of Morphology, Biochemistry, Physiology and Animal Production, Unit of Veterinary Physiology, Faculty of Veterinary Medicine, University of Messina, 98168 Messina, Italy

Take home message

A two-day-trekking event significantly affected WBC, RBC, Hb, PCV, MCHC, Plt and MCV changes in preliminary transported horses, and only RBC, Hb and PCV in untransported horses.

Lower basal WBC values and higher MCHC values were recorded in untransported horses at the 2nd day of trekking compared to preliminary transported horses.

The preliminary transport stress induced additional significant changes in variables of the haematological pattern of horses after trekking.

Introduction

The performance of a horse during competitive and not competitive events is the result of a combination of many complex interactions (Ferlazzo and Fazio, 1997; Nogueira *et al.*, 2002; Ferlazzo *et al.*, 2007; 2009), including competition experience and effects of previous transport (Fazio *et al.*, 2008a; b).

Trekking is not a competitive event, but it involves significant energy expenditure, as suggested by endocrine and haematochemical changes (Alberghina *et al.*, 2001; Medica, personal communication). Few data has been published on the haematological changes during trekking (Aronica *et al.*, 2003).

The purpose of this study was to investigate the effects of preliminary transport before trekking on haematological changes of horses during a two-day-trekking event.

Materials and methods

Twenty-nine healthy horses, aged 4 to 15 years, habitually used for trekking events were studied. The horses were individually fed on 4 kg of hay ration in the morning and in the evening, and 3 kg of bran and a commercial concentrate at 12:00 a.m; they also had free access to water.

Twenty-four of the horses (group I: 9 Thoroughbred, 5 females, 1 stallion, 3 geldings, aged 10.00±4.25; 4 Appaloosas, 1 female, 3 geldings, aged 9.33±3.79; 11 crossbred, 3 females, 2 stallions, 6 geldings, aged 11.2±4.51) were transported over distances of 70 km the day before trekking. The other five horses (group II: 5 crossbred, 1 female, 4 geldings, aged 9.25±4.19) were stabled at the starting place. Horses were weighed the day before the trekking and at the end of the two-day-trekking event on an electronic scale.

Blood samples from the jugular vein were drawn using vacutainer tubes containing EDTA (mg/ml blood) after arrival of the horses to the starting place at 04:00 p.m. the day before trekking; at 08:30 a.m. and 05:30 p.m. before and after the 1st day of trekking (length of route: 40 km, duration of trekking: 6 h, mean speed: 7 km/h; with a pause from 14:00 p.m. to 16:00 p.m. for watering the horses); at 08:30 a.m. and 1:30 p.m. before and after the 2nd day of trekking (length of route: 28 km, duration of trekking: 4 h, mean of speed: 7 km/h; without a pause for watering the horses). All samples were collected by the same operator under quiet conditions. All methods and procedures used in this study were reviewed and approved by the Messina University Institutional Board for the Care and Use of Animals.

The venous blood samples were analyzed (within 1 h) by an automatic photometer SLIM for haematological assays (SEAC) measuring White Blood Cells (WBC), Red Blood Cells (RBC), Platelets, Haemoglobin (Hb), Packed Cell Volume (PCV), Mean Corpuscular Volume (MCV), Mean Corpuscular Haemoglobin (MCH), Mean Corpuscular Haemoglobin Concentration (MCHC), Red Blood Cells Distribution Width (RDW), Mean Platelets Volume (MPV), Plateletocrit (Pct), Platelets Distribution Width (PDW).

Statistical analysis was done with a one-way repeated measures analysis of variance (RM-ANOVA) to determine whether trekking and transport had effects. Significant differences between basal and post trekking values were established using the Student's paired *t*-test. Significant differences between different groups were established using the Student's unpaired *t*-test. The level of significance was set at $P<0.05$. All calculations were performed using the PRISM package (GraphPad Software Inc., San Diego, CA, USA).

Results

Data are presented as mean ± standard deviation (mean±SD) in Table 1. As compared to basal values, statistical analyses showed significant differences between the two groups, with higher WBC and Plt values in group I after the 1st day of trekking; higher RBC and Hb in group I after the 1st and the 2nd day of trekking; higher PCV values both in group I after the 1st ($P<0.001$) and the

Table 1. Haematological variables (mean ± SD) in transported (group I) and untransported (group II) horses during a two-day-trekking event.

	Day before trekking	1st day of trekking		2nd day of trekking	
		Basal	After	Basal	After
Group I					
WBC (thousands/μl)	8.46±1.58	7.98±1.15	13.08±1.64***	10.43±2.60	12.99±2.88
RBC (millions/μl)	7.59±0.90	8.06±0.89	9.46±0.97***	7.73±1.21	9.63±1.56***
Plt (thousands/μl)	131±24	173±30	200±32*	170±25	180±48
Hb (g/dl)	12.44±1.72	13.39±1.48	15.79±1.78***	12.73±2.06	16.31±2.74***
PCV (%)	37.32±1.58	40.13±1.15	47.91±1.22***	38.79±2.60	50.33±2.10***
MCH (g/dl)	49.21±2.72	49.82±2.01	50.71±2.54	50.00±2.62	52.25±2.72**
MCV (fl)	16.37±0.92	16.62±0.79	16.69±0.86	16.45±0.78	16.94±0.93*
MCHC (g/dl)	33.34±0.25	33.36±0.45	32.95±0.35**	32.87±0.46	32.39±0.46**
RDW (%)	17.56±0.63	17.64±0.53	17.70±0.54	17.73±0.62	18.04±0.85
MPV (fl)	7.40±0.18	8.69±0.40	8.38±0.75	8.45±0.55	8.98±0.60
Pct (%)	0.10±0.02	0.15±0.03	0.17±0.04	0.14±0.03	0.16±0.04
PDW (%)	9.79±0.24	12.91±0.98	12.35±1.71	12.31±1.28	12.71±1.17
Group II					
WBC (thousands/μl)	6.95±2.19	7.51±3.55	12.40±4.24	7.63±2.10••	10.08±3.03
RBC (millions/μl)	7.62±1.41	7.52±2.21	9.03±0.66	6.77±0.73	8.05±0.93**
Plt (thousands/μl)	106±46	168±66	156±11	161±42	178±29
Hb (g/dl)	12.65±2.62	12.44±5.44	15.30±1.13	11.23±1.17	13.78±1.66**
PCV (%)	37.75±2.19	36.55±6.64	46.00±4.24*	33.80±2.88	41.77±3.03**
MCH (g/dl)	49.50±2.12	49.61±4.54	51.00±1.41	49.75±1.71	52.00±2.45**
MCV (fl)	16.55±0.49	16.52±2.21	17.00±0.02	16.60±0.64	17.08±0.49*
MCHC (g/dl)	33.50±0.28	33.31±2.14	33.35±0.78	33.28±0.31	32.93±0.48•
RDW (%)	17.10±0.14	17.51±1.98	17.60±0.14	17.53±0.34	17.95±0.42
MPV (fl)	7.30±0.14	8.55±1.87	8.65±0.07	8.23±0.71	9.43±0.78
Pct (%)	0.08±0.03	0.14±0.09	0.14±0.01	0.13±0.04	0.17±0.04
PDW (%)	10.10±0.28	11.90±2.84	13.05±0.49	11.75±1.63	14.10±0.74

WBC= White Blood Cells; RBC= Red Blood Cell; Plt= Platelets; Hb=Haemoglobin; PCV= Packed Cell Volume; MCH= Mean Corpuscular Haemoglobin; MCV=Mean Corpuscular Volume; MCHC= Mean Corpuscular Haemoglobin Concentration; RDW= Red Blood Cell Distribution Width; MPV= Mean Platelet Volume; Pct= Plateletocrit; PDW= Plateletocrit Distribution Width.

vs Basal: **P*<0.05; ***P*<0.01; ****P*<0.001. *vs* group I: •*P*<0.05; ••*P*<0.01

2nd (P<0.001) day and in group II after the 1st (P<0.05) and the 2nd (P<0.01) day of trekking; higher MCV and MCH in group II after the 2nd (P<0.05) day of trekking; lower MCHC in group I after the 1st (P<0.01) and the 2nd (P<0.01) day of trekking.

As compared to transported horses (group I), untransported horses (group II) showed basal WBC values lower (P<0.01) and MCHC values higher (P<0.05) at the 2nd day of trekking.

RM-ANOVA showed that trekking significantly affected WBC, RBC, Hb, PCV and MCHC (P<0.001), Plt (P<0.05) and MCV (P<0.01) changes in transported horses (group I), and only on RBC, Hb (P<0.05) and PCV (P<0.01) changes in untransported horses (group II).

The horses averaged 400±20 kg body weight the day before trekking and 380±10 kg at the end of the two-day-trekking event. No significant differences were observed between decreases of body weight of groups I and II.

Discussion

Data obtained showed that basal haematological values are in agreement with ranges observed in normal horses (Blood and Studdert, 2005).

The increases in haematological variables after trekking confirm previous data observed in horses after exercise (Wickler and Anderson, 2000; Hess *et al.*, 2005; Nostell *et al.*, 2006) and particularly after trekking (Aronica *et al.*, 2003). Moreover, the significant effect of trekking both in transported and untransported horses on the RBC, Hb and PCV changes suggests that these variables could be related to a response to sources of stress, like transport and exercise, and might be useful in assessing the severity of a preliminary transport stress associated with exercise.

The significantly highest WBC values in transported horses in basal condition before the 2nd day of trekking suggest that the recovery before exercise was inadequate; hence, it can be hypothesized that WBC increases were more exacerbated by exercise and could contribute to signs of muscle fatigue. These data confirm a significant post-exercise leukocytosis and the so-called 'stress leukogram' (Robson *et al.*, 2003; Krumrych, 2009), but suggest that this condition could occur when horses have not completely recovered. On the contrary, the low MCHC values after the 2nd day of trekking in transported horses showed that the effort suffered during exercise by subjects of group I was probably more than that suffered by untransported subjects (group II).

In addition, the significant increase of WBC, RBC, Plt, Hb, PCV and decrease of MCHC variables in transported horses after the 1st day of trekking could be related to the differentiated skeletal muscle effort experienced during transport and trekking. These data showed that the preliminary transport stress induced additional significant changes of haematological responses in horses after the 1st day of trekking. In addition, the compensatory time of 16 h after a transport and before trekking was probably inadequate for a complete functional recovery. Hence, when inadequate stress transport is applied and recovery time is insufficient, performance reduction could occur.

On the other hand, the significant increases of RBC, Hb, PCV, MCH and MCV variables both in group I and in group II after the 2nd day of trekking could be related to skeletal muscle effort, irrespective of the preliminary effect of transport.

The effect of haematological rhythms was not considered, because blood samples were not collected regularly over a 24 h period.

This study provides important information on the effects of length of trekking and of preliminary transport related to haematological variables that may influence the performance of horses.

References

Alberghina, A., Medica, P. and Fazio, E. (2001). In: Mester, J., King, G., Strüder, H., Tsolakidis, E., Osterburg, A. (eds.) Proc. 6th Ann. Congr. Europ. College Sport Sci., Cologne, Germany, p. 902.

Andrews, F.M., Geiger, D.R., White, S.L., Williamson, L.H., Maykuth, P.L., Green, E.M. (1995). Equine vet. J. Suppl., 20, 57-63.

Aronica, V., Medica, P., Fazio, E., Calabrò, G., Ferlazzo, A. (2003). Atti SO.F.I.VET., V, 77-78.

Blood, D.C., Studdert, V.P. (2005). In: Saunders, W.B. (ed.) Le Point Vétérinaire Italie SRL. p. 1151.

Fazio, E., Medica, P., Aronica, V., Grasso, L. Ferlazzo, A. (2008a). Acta Vet. Scand., 50, 6.

Fazio, E., Medica, P., Cravana, C., Ferlazzo, A. (2008b). Vet. Rec., 163, 713-716.

Ferlazzo, A., Fazio, E. (1997). Endocrinological variables in blood and plasma. In: A. Lindner (Ed.) Performance diagnosis of horses, Wageningen Pers, Wageningen, The Netherlands, pp. 30-43.

Ferlazzo, A., Medica, P., Fazio, E. (2007). Hormonas y Ejercicio. In: F. Boffi (Ed.) Fisiologia del Ejercicio en Equinos, Inter-Médica SAICI, Buenos Aires, República Argentina, pp.153-164.

Ferlazzo, A., Medica, P., Cravana, C., Fazio, E. (2009). Comp. Exercise Physiol., 6, 59-66.

Hargreaves, B.J., Kronfeld, D.S., Waldron, J.N., Lopes, M.A., Gay, L.S., Saker, K.E., Cooper, W.L., Sklan, D.J. Harris, P.A. (2002). Equine Vet. J., 34, 116-121.

Hess, T.M., Kronfeld, D.S., Williams, C.A., Waldron, J.N., Graham-Thiers, P.M., Greiwe-Crandell, K., Lopes, M.A., Harris, P.A. (2005). Am. J. Vet. Res., 66, 466-473.

Hoffman, R.M., Hess, T.M., Williams, C.A., Kronfeld, D.S., Griewe-Crandell, K.M., Waldron, J.E., Graham-Thiers, P.M., Gay, L.S., Splan, R.K., Saker, K.E., Harris, P.A. (2002). Equine vet. J. Suppl., 34, 39-43.

Jablonska, E.M., Ziolkowska, S.M., Gill, J., Szykula, R., Faff, J. (1991). Equine vet. J., 23, 309-311.

Krumrych, W. (2009). Bull. Vet. Inst. Pulawy, 53, 97-103.

Nogueira, G.P., Barnabe, R.C., Bedran-de-Castro, J.C., Moreira, A.F., Fernandes, W.R., Mirandola, R.M.S., Howard, D.L. (2002). Braz. J. Vet. Res. Anim. Sci., 39, 54-57.

Nostell, K., Funkquist, P., Nyman, G., Essén-Gustavsson, B., Connysson, M., Muhonen, S., Jansson, A. (2006). Equine vet. J. Suppl., 36, 123-127.

Robson, P.J., Alston, T.D., Myburgh, K.H. (2003). Equine Vet. J., 35, 133-137.

Sommardahl, C.S., Andrews, F.M., Saxton, A.M., Geiser, D.R., Maykuth, P.L. (1994). Am. J. Vet. Res., 55, 389-394.

Wickler, S.J., Anderson, T.P. (2000). Am. J. Physiol. Regul. Integr. Comp. Physiol., 279, R1176-R1181.

Williamson, L.H., Andrews, F.M., Maykuth, P.L., White, S.L., Green, E.M. (1996). Equine vet. J., Suppl., 22, 92-98.

Williams C.A., Kronfeld, D.S., Hess, T.M., Saker, K.E., Waldron, J.N., Crandell, K.M., Hoffman, R.M., Harris, P.A. (2004). J. Anim. Sci., 82, 588-594.

Wood, S.C., Fedde, M.R. (1997). Respir. Physiol.,107, 165-172.

Practical experience on what the good performer requires

Philippe Benoit[1] (Showjumping), Anne Couroucé-Malblanc[2] (3day), Chris E. Kawcak[3] (Western Riding), Brian D. Nielsen[4], E. Hank Bird[5] (THB racehorse) and Marianne M. Sloet van Oldruitenborgh-Oosterbaan[6] (Endurance)
[1]*Clinique Equine, 4 Route de Vilpert, 78610 Les Breviares, France*
[2]*ONIRIS (Ecole Nationale Vétérinaire, Agroalimentaire et de l'Alimentation de Nantes Atlantique), Unité de médecine, Atlanpôle – La Chantrerie, 44307 Nantes cedex, France; anne.courouce@oniris-nantes.fr*
[3]*Equine Orthopaedic Research Center, Colorado State University, 300 West Drake Rd, Fort Collins, CO 80523, USA*
[4]*Michigan State University, East Lansing, MI 48824, USA*
[5]*Steephollow Farm, Bryan, TX 77808, USA*
[6]*Department of Equine Sciences, Faculty of Veterinary Medicine, Utrecht University, Yalelaan 114, 3584 CM Utrecht, the Netherlands*

Introduction

Athletic horses may perform in various disciplines such as races (gallop, trot, endurance) or sport disciplines (showjumping, 3-day-event, dressage, western riding, ...). Performance is multifactorial and is based on physical qualities (conformation of the horse, locomotor system), physiological qualities (cardiovascular, respiratory, muscular, systems) and also mental qualities. One horse may perform in one discipline but may not be a good performer in another one. Therefore, a good performer may require various qualities according to the discipline. The practical experience of different authors will be detailed in this paper with a focus on showjumping, 3-day-event, western riding, gallop and endurance racing.

The high level show jumper

In order to share a practical experience on what the high level jumper requires, I will write about the pre purchase exam as it is a very specific type of examination which aim is to determine if a particular horse is able to participate in high level competition as a jumper.

- The horse has to be sound to compete at the expected level.
- The horse needs to have a good physical exam and musculoskeletal status if needed to be sold.
- The horse with its potential problem will have to be managed in a certain environment that we need to evaluate too (stabling, training, footing, shoeing…).

The challenge is to assess a horse of which we have no or limited prior knowledge. Our goal as vet practitioners will be to evaluate the risk and give our client a way of managing the horse after the decision of purchase. This will end up as a more detailed and specific type of exam. We will go through all the steps of a conventional exam adding specific tests and enquiries that should be evaluated to give a final comment to the potential buyer.

History of the horse

The practitioner will have to make like an enquiry to get a maximum amount of information in a small amount of time.

If possible:

- Communicating with other professionals who have had prior dealings with horse: the veterinarian, the farrier, the physiotherapist, the trainer, the rider.
- Accessing to previous clinical records, medical images, videos.
- Finding competition records and check dates to see if there are gaps of time in between suspecting rest or injuries.
- Trying to know what the horse has been living with.

Looking at the passport:

- Check vaccination record in agreement with national law and FEI rules.
- Check number and frequency of show the horse participated to.
- For ponies, make sure that the withers height is correct under National or FEI rules.

Static exam

- Medical / internal part: heart auscultation has to be rigorous even if most of the heart pathologies (exception of major heart rhythm pathologies as atrial fibrillation) are well tolerated in the jumper. Special care of the lung auscultation should be done since a few diseases including EIPH (use of endoscopy and potential Xrays) are definitely affecting performance. Upper respiratory problems such as roaring are affecting partially the condition but would be a challenge in case of resale.
- Teeth evaluation is part of most of the behaviour induced problems which are underestimated, and may interfere with source of neck, back pain and misbehaviour
- Orthopaedic / conformation: there have been a few attempts to find a relation between physical conformation and ability of jumping with poor success. Nevertheless, there are a few findings we prefer not to have for the high level competition:

1. Extreme defect of front feet weight bearing (toe in or toe out) and long pastern low fetlock axis on front or hinds as they are known to promote a real risk of suspensory ligament strain and lesion.
2. Muscling should be as symmetric as possible. Special observation will be given to base of withers, low neck and especially gluteus area.
3. Some joints may be mildly effusive with no significant clinical relation unless passive flexion tests are positive (painful as the horse is standing).

Dynamic exam

As usual, the dynamic exam starts on a straight line and on a figure 8 at the walk where maximum attention is given to the way the horse bends sideways and the axial skeleton should align itself naturally to the curve. This will give ideas of any areas of defect of motion between the top of the neck to the tail. Each fetlock should drop (overextend) equally. At the trot on straight line and circles, the horse is examined with special interest to the back motion which should be evaluated sideways and from behind. For sure any source of discomfort, including defect of cranial phase or caudal phase of the stride will be noticed.

High level jumpers may show extraordinary length of stride, and some hyperextension of the front / hind limbs movement that should be differentiated from moderate uncoordination.

On the circle, again, same attention is given to bending at trot and canter. Every part of the body should move fluently as a 'wave'. The canter should be a good 3 beat with nice suspension phase. The horse should remain perpendicular to the ground on a lunge line and not leaning inside (more characteristic of lumbosacral type of pain). The horse can be sound but having trouble to maintain a nice equivalent and symmetric stride from one side to the other. Therefore, a horse that does not hold the lead, counter canters, or has a moderate dissociation of both hinds might be suspected of having hind limb subclinical problems that may not show up in a conventional exam.

The surcingle test (Desbrosse) gives a good idea of potential thoracic pain or longissimus spasms.

Dynamic flexion tests are mandatory and should be negative for most of this high level sport horses. A comparison of the weight and ease to flex should be contrasted with the findings of the static exam to evaluate potential improvement due to the warm up.

Dynamic hoof test is systematically done in our practice to underline any source of local heel pain as the horse jogs (even more significant when a horse showed a shorter stride circling on hard footing).

Exam under tack

Such high level horses should be seen under tack. This involves two challenges: (1) asking the horse to be ridden by another person than the official rider; (2) having a professional insurance cover this type of demand, which is not widely accepted. But, this exam is in our opinion, a very interesting exam to pick up subtle lameness or defect of symmetry when changing reins. This exercise may help to understand subtle abnormality that the horse may exacerbate once he competes at the highest level.

The protocol is always the same having the horse in a light frame on a large figure 8 at the trot, and the rider is asked to change lead of diagonal to see the change in the weight bearing of each 4 limbs. We found per example this test very relevant to pick up early stifle or suspensory source of discomfort as the rider is loading with the inside limb (fore or hind).

For the same purpose, it is very interesting to watch videos of the horse performing and note any source of abnormality such as:

- Landing on a preferred limb.
- Defect of bending of one part of the back between fences or over the fence.
- Defect of canter stride (length, disunited, gait) from left to right.
- Difficulty to collect in between fences.

After dynamic exam, I am willing to palpate and manipulate the back, neck, flexor tendons and major joints to look for any source of pain, distension and differences with my earlier findings when the horse was cold and standing.

All the information collected after this full clinical examination should lead to list the good and bad points of the horse itself and try to make a hierarchy of problems according to the type of discipline.

At this stage, even if imaging including at least Xrays and ultrasound exams are done, there is a need to make sure, especially for older horses to understand that abnormal findings on the clinical exam and imaging techniques should be matching so the practitioner can give at least a potential diagnosis but also a prognosis when possible. This again will put the practitioner in a more critical position where he may advice a follow up procedure to maintain the horse in the sport.

Xray exam

Most of the normal Xray check ups have been already described in many lectures. There are a few possibilities to create a standard amount of pictures. Our aim again is to obtain a maximum amount of information with a minimum of Xrays. In most of these check up I may prefer to have views of the neck, back, and splint bones to confirm or document my clinical exam instead of always repeating the conventional ratio of Xray images.

From the standard protocol involving all the distal joints, I may certainly ask for low neck and mid back Xrays, which could be completed with ultrasound imaging.

Ultrasonography

This type of imaging should be done each time the horse is more than 7 years old and already competes at high level. Younger horses, also depending of the amount of transaction, should be considered to have at least a base line of some ligament and tendon structures. We normally examine the following structures:

- Suspensory ligament (proximal area) on 4 limbs almost systematically.
- Suspensory distal branches, SDFT and fetlock ligaments especially on long pastern low fetlock conformation horses.
- Neck cervical epiaxial joints evaluation on stiff neck horses, or showing light uncoordination.
- Back: Thoraco-lumbar area and epiaxial lumbar joints externally, and if pelvis motion is poor and if both parties agree, I would propose internal rectal evaluation of sacro-iliac and lumbosacral joints.

Endoscopy

When vetting high level performers in show jumping, it is quiet easy to have access to videos or trials of the client or usual rider. Therefore, if the horse is a roarer or shows abnormal noise during exercise, it will be easy to have a quick information and make an upper respiratory tract endoscopy to document this noise. Therefore, if the horse has not shown such pathology and has a normal slap test, I may not, after asking my client and making my own assessment, follow up with an endoscopy. This also means at the contrary, that abnormal finding, including respiratory auscultation, should lead the practitioner to make an endoscopy.

Gastroscopy

This type of exam is even more invasive than the previous type of endoscopy. Therefore, it will be never done on a systematic base. We should try to have enough information from previous owner and professionals working with the horse to know if the horse has been suffering from gastritis and/or ulcers. This disease appears to be significantly responsible of many counter performance issues and we see in our experience horses suffering from chronic back pain with related gastritis. Subsequently, I may try to obtain the authorization from owner to do this exam in the near future (before transaction) if there is any high suspicion during the pre purchase clinical exam.

This is one of this exam that you may ask to be done as complementary to document a clinical suspicion and give your client maximum information before the final transaction.

Other type of imaging

MRI and Bone Scan have been already done in a few scenarios of pre purchase exam. There is nevertheless a barrier to be established to avoid such exams, unless the practitioner needs very precise information to help his client making a very fine decision. When it comes to such exam, it is more to fail the horse, which most of the vets can definitely do by doing a very thorough clinical exam and therefore avoid undertaking this type of medical imaging.

I would consider essentially the case of a horse which has been injured, and comes for sale with a good documentation, eventually with MRI images, that may need such an imaging to track or prove a specific healing process or the stabilisation of a known lesion (bone oedema, cartilage thinning, ligament strain…) before the decision for transaction.

Blood work

High level jumpers are subject to travel far from home, and may also be resold in foreign countries where certain serology must be negative.

- For all of them, I will ask for a Coggins test.
- For stallion and high potential mares, I may propose my clients to do a CEM swap.
- For any other horses, especially travelling, or sold to USA and competing overseas, you must do a piroplasmosis serology in an appropriate laboratory.
- Finally, we run systematically a blood cell count and a standard biochemistry.

- Medication test are also done on whole blood, even if we are aware that we will pick up only recent use of drugs, and this test will include anti-inflammatory drugs, sedatives, bronchodilatators and steroids.

Conclusion

The pre purchase exam of the high level jumper is like a police enquiry which starts with the collection of a great amount of information around the history, and performance record of the horse. The practitioner, besides doing a normal standard exam, shall go in some more specific clinical tests and imaging procedures to document some of the most challenging patterns that are difficult to manage.

Our role is to identify the good and poor sides of the horse in order to maintain the horse in the sport, or to be sold again if we are dealing with professional riders or dealers. Therefore, it becomes a challenge to list the problems of the horse giving our own hierarchy to be able to offer a very individual and specific management. This shall be done in agreement with our knowledge of the future rider and professional environment, which includes the stabling, the training, and all the individuals working as a team with the vet practitioner.

References

Andrews, J. (2005) Gastric ulcers in horses. J Anim Sci 83: 18-21.

Benoit, P. (2006) How to make a specific examination of the jumper. In: Proc Am Assoc Eq Pract, San Antonio.

Boswell, R., Mitchell, R., Dyson, S. (2003) Lameness in the show hunter and show jumper. In: Ross MW and Dyson SJ, eds. Diagnosis and Management of Lameness in the Horse, St. Louis: Saunders. Pp 965-975.

Château, H., Degeurce, C., Denoix, J.M. (2005) Influence de la nature du sol et de la ferrure sur la biomécanique des articulations digitales. In: Proc 31ème journée de la Recherche Equine: 35-44.

Denoix, J.M. (1999) Spinal biomechanics and functional anatomy. Vet Clin North Am: 15: 27-60.

Denoix, J.M. (2008) Biomecanique du cheval de CSO. In: Proc Assoc Vét Eq Française.

Denoix, J.M., Dyson, S.J. (2003) The thoracolumbar spine. In: Ross MR and Dyson SJ, eds. Diagnosis and lameness in Horses. Saint Louis, WB Saunders. Pp 509-521.

Dyson, S., Benoit, P. (2008) Monitoring orthopaedic health in competition horses. In: The acute poorly performing sport horses – CESMAS. Wageningen Academic Publishers, Wageningen, the Netherlands, p91-94.

Jeffcott, L.B. (1980) Disorders of the thoracolumbar spine of the horse – a survey of 443 cases. Eq Vet J 12: 197-210.

Mitchell, R.D. (2001) Prevalence of gastric ulcers in hunter/jumper and dressage horses evaluated for poor performance. In: Proc Association for Equine Sports Medicine.

The high level Three-Day-Event horse

Eventing consists of three different disciplines: 1) dressage which is a test of discipline and precision; 2) cross country which is a test of power, strength, stamina and bravery of horse and rider; 3) show-jumping which is a test of accuracy.

All sorts of horses compete successfully up to novice level. However, to go on beyond novice level, a horse with a fair amount of natural athletic ability is required. A horse's ability and mental aptitude are the most important determinants (Bathe, 2003). Until now, many of the top level event horses have been full or three-quarter Thoroughbred and many of these have not been big horses. Often medium height horses are easier to manoeuvre and can more easily negotiate difficult distances or turns. Small, lean looking horses usually have excellent bone circumference to bodyweight ratios, and stand up well to hard and fast work. The most common types of injuries in event horses are soft tissue injuries such as tendon and ligament damage. When selecting youngsters to compete in eventing, it pays to select those individuals with good conformation in order to avoid putting any unnecessary strain on the connective tissue structures of the distal limb (Marlin, 2005). The financial value of event horses is considerably lower than that for racehorses, show jumpers or dressage horses so any horse with outstanding ability in one of these phases is likely to be used in that sport first. If the horse does not succeed, then they may be tried as potential event horses. These horses bring with them any injuries they may have accumulated, but because of the different stresses imposed during eventing, this may not be a problem. For example, event horses tolerate low-grade carpal pathological conditions from previous race training (Bathe, 2003). A small number of horses are bred specifically for eventing. Stallions are generally considered to lack the courage required to compete at the top level. In the UK, geldings continue to be the most popular choice for eventing, with their use increasing with grade (Marlin, 2005).

Physical demands of eventing

The FEI star system is designed so that there should be a progressive increase in difficulty when moving from one-star up to four-star competitions. Certainly for the cross-country phase this is usually the case (Schroter and Marlin, 2002). Whilst the size of the jumps and the number of obstacles are similar for all one-day or three-day events within a certain class of competition, events vary considerably in terms of the physiological demands they place on a horse. Some cross-country courses are on near flat terrain, whilst others involve steep uphill and downhill gradients (Schroter and Marlin, 2002). Firm going may predispose to lameness in some horses, whilst soft going (after rain or even sand) can increase the effort by up to 30% and may also cause muscle and tendon injuries.

Most competing horses have natural cross ability. They are also selected for natural jumping action, but jumping technique during the cross country is different than that needed for show jumping. The event horse's weakest link is usually the dressage phase as the different breeding and level of fitness of these horses mean that the major challenge can be to control the horse's temperament.

For eventing, the basic conformation of the horse must be correct as it is unforgiving to conformational defects compared with show jumping and dressage. The general principles are the same as for any equine athlete. Serious conformational defects include being back at the knee, having upright pasterns and hocks and a moderate or severe toed-out conformation. Of slightly lesser significance are a long or short back, being over at the knee, or having long sloping pasterns (Bathe, 2003).

Physiological demands of eventing

Dressage Phase

There is very little published on the physiology of the horse in response to Dressage competition in one or three-day events, or even in pure Dressage. Following a mean warm-up time of 58 min, horses performing a preliminary level dressage test in a one-star three-day event in thermally stressful conditions (WBGT index ~33 °C) had a mean heart rate of 92±5 bpm (Marlin *et al.*, 2001). This compares with a mean heart rate of 103±14 bpm for horses performing an elementary level test in pure Dressage in cool conditions. Heart rates for horses performing collected trot at Grand Prix are reported to be in the range of 80-100 bpm and 120-140 bpm for half-pass (Clayton, personal communication).

Cross-country test

Considerably more information exists concerning the physiological demands of cross-country either in one-day or three-day events, however there is currently no published information on the demands of the short-format CIC test. Heart rate is an acceptable indicator of exercise intensity. The mean heart rates published in the scientific literature for horses competing in Horse Trials range from 155 (1*) to 195 bpm (4*) (Kohn and Hinchcliff, 1995; Kohn *et al.*, 1995; Marlin *et al.*, 1995; White *et al.*, 1995a; White *et al.*, 1995b).

The data for heart rate during cross-country shows that the intensity of exercise increases with increasing level, and that this is most marked for horse-trials.

Show-jumping

As for the dressage phase, there is minimal published information on the heart rate of horses during the show-jumping phase of eventing. Following a mean duration of warm-up of 38±30 min and at a WBGT index of ~31 °C, the mean heart rate of horses undertaking show-jumping in a one-star three-day event was 147±6 bpm (Marlin *et al.*, 2001). Heart rates in horses competing in the Belgian Junior Show-Jumping Championships were reported to be 178±5 bpm and 191±4 bpm, at the start and end of the course, respectively (Art *et al.*, 1990). In the study of event horses jumping, jump heights were 1.1 metres (Marlin *et al.*, 2001), whilst in the study of Art *et al.* (1990) the fences were 1.5 metres high, which may explain the higher heart rates.

Eventing is a discipline for which horses should be complete athletes. These horses should have intrinsic physical and physiological qualities which may be developed with training. At high level, monitoring the training of these horses is of great importance in order to develop their qualities while preventing injuries.

References

Art, T., Amory, H., Desmecht, D., Lekeux, P. (1990) Effect of show jumping on heart rate, blood lactate and other plasma biochemical values. Eq Vet J Suppl, 78-82.

Bathe, A.P. (2003) Lameness in the Three Day Event Horse. In: Diagnosis abd management of lameness in the horse. Ross, M.W., Dyson, S.J. (eds.), Saunders. Pp 984-995.

Clayton, H.M. (1997) Effect of added weight on landing kinematics in jumping horses. Eq Vet J Suppl, 50-53.

Kohn, C.W., Hinchcliff, K.W. (1995) Physiological responses to the endurance test of a 3-day-event during hot and cool weather. Eq Vet J Suppl, 31-36.

Kohn, C.W., Hinchcliff, K.W., McCutcheon, L.J., Geor, R., Foreman, J., Allen, A.K., White, S.L., Maykuth, P.L., Williamson, L.H. (1995) Physiological responses of horses competing at a modified 1 star 3-day-event. Eq Vet J Suppl, 97-104.

Marlin, D.J., Harris, P.A., Schroter, R.C., Harris, R.C., Roberts, C.A., Scott, C.M., Orme, C.E., Dunnett, M., Dyson, S.J., Barrelet, F. *et al.* (1995) Physiological, metabolic and biochemical responses of horses competing in the speed and endurance phase of a CCI*****3-day-event. Eq Vet J Suppl, 37-46.

Marlin, D.J., Schroter, R.C., Mills, P.C., White, S.L., Maykuth, P.L., Votion, D., Waran, N. (2001) Performance of acclimatized european horses in a modified one star (*) three-day event in heat and humidity. J Eq Vet Sci 21, 341-350.

Marlin, D.J. (2005) In: Proceeding of AVEF, Angers.

Schroter, R.C., Marlin, D.J. (2002) Modelling the oxygen cost of transport in competitions over ground of variable slope. Eq Vet J Suppl, 397-401.

White, S.L., Williamson, L.H., Maykuth, P.L., Cole, S.P., Andrews, F.M. (1995a) Heart rate response and plasma lactate concentrations of horses competing in the speed and endurance phase of 3-day combined training events. Eq Vet J Suppl, 52-56.
White, S.L., Williamson, L.H., Maykuth, P.L., Cole, S.P., Andrews, F.M., Geiser, D.R. (1995b) Heart rate response and plasma lactate concentrations of horses competing in the cross-country phase of combined training events. Eq Vet J Suppl, 47-51.

The high level Western Riding horse

The American Quarter Horse was developed as a breed in the 1600's by the American colonists who crossed English Thoroughbred type horses with horses that were native to the Americas at that time. These latter horses were from Spanish, Arabian and Barb stock and brought to North America by the Spanish. This resulted in a relatively small but hardy and quick breed of horse (Scott, 2008). Initially these horses were found to be rather fast in a quarter mile race and were used for this purpose. However, with the westward expansion of the Americas and the development of the beef industry, the use of this breed was focused mostly on ranch work. These horses were found to be quick and agile, were patient around cattle yet aggressive in their work and developed extensive mental and physical durability. This early western work then stimulated competitive events in which horses were compared in their all around versatility as a ranch horse. Today there are over 3.2 million Quarter Horses worldwide making them the most popular breed in the world. There are several organizations that have expanded from the United States into Canada, Europe and Australia (Curry, 1997).

Western performance horses are divided into two types. The first types are those that are used in rodeo competition. Rodeos evolved from competitions between ranches in the late 1800's in which the cowboys and their horses competed to determine the most versatile individuals. Events include tie-down calf roping, team roping (divided into heading and heeling horses) and barrel racing. Tie down calf roping involves roping the calf, tying them down for general care in the field by a single individual. These horses need to be fast, have a quick effective stop and back quickly in order to allow the rider to get to the calf as quickly as possible. Heading horses used for team roping are larger in order to pull the steer. They must be very fast and strong. Heeling horses used for team roping need to have an ability to interact with the steer. This means that they can track the steer without cueing from the rider, similar to calf roping horses, and can stop effectively and back up quickly. Barrel racing was developed in the mid 1900's to compare speed and agility between ranch horses. These horses are usually of racing stock and are not only fast but can turn quickly. Overall the rodeo horses are older and more mature and their durability into their late teens is essential.

The second type of western performance horse is a stock horse which includes horses used in cutting (a technique used for separating cattle during processing and weaning) and all purpose ranch use. Some of the early all purpose events were performed by the Vaqueros in California in the 1800's as a test of the versatility of the ranch horse. Cutting horses were developed in West Texas in the late 1800's again as a method of separating cattle. Since cattle have a strong herd instinct a versatile cutting horse was essential for not only separating but keeping cattle away from the herd for processing. The horse needs to mirror the cow's movement and therefore needs to be quick, agile, intelligent and calm but aggressive. Reining horses were developed again in the late 1800's in order to show versatility in ranch work. These horses are slightly larger than cutting horses and need to be fast with long, engaging stops, the ability to perform large and tight circles and need to be calm but agile. The reined cow horse was developed in California specifically by the Vaqueros and can be considered an all purpose horse. These horses perform cutting, reining and working cow horse (which demonstrate the horse's ability to isolate a cow and manipulate it in the free range) events all within one performance. Overall these various events show the versatility of the American Quarter Horse and consequently result in a number of musculoskeletal issues depending on the event.

Some of the differences in these performance uses are due to the use itself but also the timeline for which these horses are used. The stock horses typically undergo basic training for 60-90 days starting between 18 and 24 months of age. They are taught to walk, trot and canter to stop, turn and to switch leads. After 90 days they then work with a single cow in a round pen, less than 50 meters in diameter, and learn to become engaging with the cattle. This is where the horses sense of engagement with the cattle is determined and sometimes their lack of engagement will dictate that they be used for other purposes. The horse learns to demonstrate a complete and balanced stop and during this time learns to mirror the cows movements. They are usually trained 2 to 4 days per week for 3 to 4 months. At this time the horse learns to predict the cow's movement without over-anticipating. Most trainers feel that there is a strong genetic influence on this trait (Black, 2003). The ultimate goal here is for the horse to learn to mirror the cow's movements with minimal cues from the rider. Most of the stock horse events then lead to futurities late in their 3-year-old year, usually in the fall and winter. A horse cannot have competed officially prior to entry into a futurity, and so it is their first real performance. Most of these horses will compete from the end of their 3-year-old year until the end of their 6-year-old year. After that the chance to earn money is diminished but the horses can still compete later in age at amateur events. Usually by this time there is an aggressive push for these horses to enter a breeding program since most of the money earned in the industry is through breeding and not performance.

Most stock horse events at the highest level have two elimination rounds followed by semi-finals and finals all within a few days. Consequently this places incredible physical and mental stress on the animals. However, there is a strong resurgence at these events as most of the major events will now have over 1000 entries with a total purse often times greater than the Triple Crown of Thoroughbred racing. Like other performance horses, the same horse can been shown by a professional in an open division as well as by the owner in either a non-pro or amateur division (Black, 2003). Therefore, a single horse, shown by both the professional trainer and its owner may perform upwards of 8 times within a 2 week period, again often leading to fatigue-related injuries.

Conformation evaluation of the Western Performance horse is essential especially for the different disciplines. Consequently personal experience by the veterinarian with each discipline is critical (Ross, 2003). Conformation should be evaluated both statically and dynamically. The dynamic conformation evaluation is essential because some horses can have slightly abnormal static conformation yet can be successful due to their aggressive nature, intelligence and competitiveness much as we see in humans. Overall most of these horses are 14 to 15 hands (1.42 to 1.52 m) in height although reining horses, reined cow horses, heading horses and barrel racing horses can be slightly taller. They usually have a short back, strong hips and of course correct limb conformation. As mentioned before there is a slight variation with each discipline. For calf roping, the horses are usually older and sometimes are retired cutting horses. They have a strong back and pelvis and also a strong shoulder and chest for quick, effective stopping and backing. These horses should be quite intelligent because again they need to engage with the cattle with minimal cues from the rider. Heading horses on the other hand are aggressive and fast. They are larger, have a strong shoulder, neck and pelvis in order to not only catch the steer but to then turn its entire weight for the heeler to then perform. These horses do not need to be as engaging with the steer as a calf roping and heeling horse. Heeling horses are again smaller and are sometimes ex-cutting horses. They have good engagement with the cow and a very good stop. Cutting horses are smaller, being from 14 to 15 hands in height and have to have a good effective stop that facilitates quick turns and instant acceleration. They are typically lighter in the neck but should have a good sloping shoulder for an effective turn and a strong front end for effective turning as well. Low hock conformation and strong hind end is ideal and because of their aggressive use at a young age early maturity is a positive trait. Reining horses are usually larger and fast with good balance for long stops, although they have less use of their forelimbs than some of the other disciplines. They need to be strong for the stop and agile for turning. Reined cow horses are usually taller and leaner than cutting horses and need to show incredible intelligence, maturity and durability for use in all three events. Although these are generalizations for use in the different disciplines there can be some variability. For instance, there are some very effective cutting horses that have relatively long backs however their intelligence, aggressiveness and will to win often override these minor flaws. Rodeo horses are typically older and usually more mature in their performance. However, they undergo work in incredibly variable footing and are often hauling great distances and performing numerous events in short periods of time. Therefore these horses need to have both physical and mental durability in order to withstand the rigors of work.

Conformational traits that are problematic to the Western Performance horse include both toe in and toe out conformation. These place incredible stress on the feet and the proximal suspensory ligaments and if not dealt with early can lead to loss of use. Offset knees are also a problem as they too can lead to significant stress in the proximal suspensory ligaments as well as the branches of the proximal suspensory ligament and on the fetlock joints. A short hip in the cranial caudal direction can lead to increased stress on the stifles and hocks and a lot of these horses will have a performance limiting problem just because they do not have a strong stop and the concussion of stopping can place incredible stress on those joints. However, this conformation can evolve with maturity through muscle development. Horses with a sickle hock conformation have increased stress on their hind suspensory ligaments and hocks and a narrow hock conformation or base narrow conformation in the hind limbs can place stress on the hips and the back. However, as mentioned before horses with these static conformational abnormalities should be evaluated dynamically as some of them have the mental integrity and neuromuscular control to overcome these flaws if they are minor.

Selection of the Western Performance horse sometimes depends on how the horse is raised. The dam's conformation and performance record subjectively have a large impact on selection of a young horse. The mare's performance history is a strong indicator of the mental ability and aggressiveness of the horse. Some of these mares are more apt to be bred thanks to embryo transfer during their performance years and right after. Although this quickly propagates these positive traits some of these mares are bred due to injury which may propagate negative conformational and mental problems as well. The breeder's reputation is also important. As discussed in another article in this book proper physical work at a young age is essential to strengthen musculoskeletal tissues later in life. Those foals and yearlings that are managed through stall rest are usually avoided due to weakness in the tissues later in life (Kawcak *et al.*, 2010). The breeder's perception of the individual's attitude is also important. When evaluating young horses it is good to watch them interact with their pasture mates to see if they are engaging and competitive. It is good to evaluate them individually to see if the horse, even as a yearling, will do the things you want them to do willingly such as turning in the stall and if they are engaging with people. Although controversial, some people justify evaluating foals and yearlings in a round pen to look at their dynamic conformation and engagement. Again, here the goal is to see how well the foal or yearling uses itself.

Evaluation during early training is also used for selection of Western Performance horses. Most rodeo horses are already trained and the rider has some insight on the performance capability of the individual. Most barrel racing horses are retired racehorses and consequently their ability to develop agile quick turns is essential to evaluate. Heading horses are usually used for all around use and again their quickness and durability are assessed during this time. Stock horses on the other hand undergo intense early training starting between 18 and 42 months of age. For cutting horses their intelligence and engagement with cattle becomes fairly obvious during the early training period as a 2-year-old (Black, 2003). This is similar with reining horses and reined cow horses. This is a place where assessment of intelligence is most important as a horse that is willing to work and not made to work is desirable. During this early training period minor conformational and developmental flaws can become apparent. Although most horses at the highest levels are radiographed as yearlings there are some developmental orthopedic diseases that become apparent during early training. These are aggressively treated at this time point since conservative therapy may result in the need for surgery during a 3-year-old year which is not desirable. Most of these horses are left barefoot during early training therefore foot soreness can become apparent at this time. Again, this is also a time where incorrect balance to the feet is addressed with the goal of the horse landing flat.

Selection of the Western Performance horse continues with late training and during performance. For the rodeo horse, fatigue is a problem and the determination of durability occurs during this time. Again, they work on variable footing with a lot of shipping and consequently most early problems develop as a behavioral issue. It is essential during these early behavioral changes that the horse be examined for fatigue related lameness problems. Fatigue also plays a role with stock horses later in their 3-year-old year. Stallions in particular seem to undergo significant fatigue. These horses are typically excited and sometime hard to focus. Some trainers will castrate these horses at an early age in order to alleviate this problem but if the horse shows early talent and can be justified as breeding stock he may be left intact. In these cases it is not uncommon for these easily excited horses to become sore in their backs and hips. Most problems in stock horses occur as performance limiting issues such as decrease in their ability to stop and turn and they begin to loose interest with their engagement with the cattle. At this age it is sometimes difficult to know if the veterinarian is dealing with low grade soreness or a true injury. These horses are constantly monitored every few weeks, particularly in areas such as their suspensory ligaments, stifles, hind fetlocks, backs, hips, semitendinosus and semimembranosus muscles and hocks. The hind ankles are of significant interest considering that plantar metatarsal arthrosis is not uncommon in these horses. In addition to all these musculoskeletal factors the veterinarian must be aware of stress induced problems such as gastric ulcers that are typical at this age. In addition equine protozoal myelitis (EPM) is of significant concern especially in a young, stressed horse. Often times an aggressive neurologic workup is needed in order to determine whether EPM can be an issue.

In summary, with the expansion in interest in Western Performance horses both in the US and abroad, aggressive monitoring has become standard of care for managing these athletes. Consequently more stress has been placed on selection criteria for these horses and today static and dynamic physical conformation as well as mental and behavioral components are all evaluated. Overall this is a dynamic group of horses to work on, and the veterinarian is essential for the success of these horses.

References

Scott, M. (2008) Musculoskeletal injuries in nonracing quarter horses. Vet Clin North Am Equine Pract 24, 133-152.

Curry, A.K. (1997) The Western Performance Horse. In: Proc Am Assoc Equine Pract 43, 46-48.

Black, J.B. (2003) The Cutting Horse. In: Ross, Dyson, eds. Philadelphia: Saunders. Pp 1017.

Ross, M. (2003) Diagnosis and Management of Lameness in the Horse In: Ross, Dyson, eds. Philadelphia: Saunders. Pp 15.

Kawcak, C.E., McIlwraith, C.W., Firth, E. (2010) Effects of early exercise on metacarpophalangeal joints in horses. Am J Vet Res in press 71: 405-411.

The high level Thoroughbred racehorse

It is commonly recognized that 'racehorses' can come in all shapes and sizes. Anyone who has spent a day at the track will notice that all horses that make it into the winner's circle do not look exactly alike. However, when selecting a horse for possible success on the track, experience suggests that there exist certain desirable traits, as well as others that should be avoided.

The first thing that one would want to have in a racehorse is balance. This would suggest being able to divide the horse fairly equally into thirds with the front end, middle, and hind end nearly the same length and fitting well together. Typically a relatively short, powerful back with a long underline is desired. Having a long underline allows the horse to take a longer stride, but this length needs to be balanced with a long neck, useful for balance, and a long hip for power in the hind end. A 2:1 underline:topline ratio is desirable, which also corresponds to a 2:1 crest of the neck:underside of neck ratio for optimal balance. A horse should be deep through the girth as heartgirth circumference has been positively correlated with win percentage (Smith *et al.*, 2006). This depth through the heartgirth should carry back through the flank to avoid the look of being 'waspy-waisted'. Such horses tend to be higher in the croup and are longer in the loin and weaker in the coupling. A balanced horse would typically be as deep in the girth as it is long in the legs. In an unbalanced horse, one usually finds a shallow girth, resulting in the appearance of longer legs.

One advantage of being deep in the heartgirth is to allow for greater respiratory capacity. Being able to breathe easily is a critical aspect of being able to perform well. A large nostril suggests a greater ability to take in large amounts of air, though this relationship has not been well documented. Many trainers place their hands or fists underneath the mandible of a horse to determine the intermandibular width. Some research supports the idea that a greater intermandibular width is related to improved performance (Cator, 1991; Cook, 1988; Delahunty *et al.*, 1991), however, a study examining over 3,000 Thoroughbreds reported a small inverse relationship between mature intermandibular width and highest racing performance. Interestingly, when comparing the mature height of a horse to its intermandibular width, a greater percentage of graded stakes winners had a more narrow intermandibular width relative to their height (Mostert and Householder, 2000) suggesting that the width may be more reflective of body type. Wide-bodied individuals that have greater intermandibular width may be more suited for sprint racing while the narrower intermandibular width may reflect a horse better suited for distance racing. Thus, intermandibular width appears to be of only limited use in predicting racing potential.

Often horses undergo an endoscopic examination before a sale to determine if there are respiratory issues, but sometimes too much emphasis is placed on the results of such an examination. Obviously, if there is a tremendous amount of airway occlusion due to laryngeal hemiplegia, that horse should probably be avoided. Sometimes horses are removed from consideration when there is some swelling of the arytenoid cartilage that may only be temporary. However, when a horse has laryngeal hemiplegia and 'roars,' there is a reduction in peak inspiratory airflow and increased inspiratory impedance. When the left recurrent laryngeal nerve, the longest nerve in the body, fails to innervate the left cricoarytenoideus dorsalis muscle of the larynx, 'roaring' develops (Jones, 1993). There is some belief that this may be more common in horses selected for long necks (Brakenhoff *et al.*, 2006). Though having a long neck is important for good balance and contributes to an attractive appearance, it is possible for a horse's neck to be too long. This may result in impaired air intake if issues with the left laryngeal nerve develop. Thus, while a long neck is desirable, especially when compared to a short neck, there is a limit as to how long one would want it. Besides anatomical characteristics that contribute to air intake, having good air quality in the horse's home environment is vitally important for performance. Granted, this is something easier to control once a horse is owned as compared to something one can evaluate when one is looking to purchase.

While depth of the chest is important, having a wide chest floor between the front legs may not be as crucial. Though useful in horses that perform many lateral movements, such as cutting horses, a wide chest floor is often indicative of having a greater proportion of fast twitch fibers. Thoroughbred racehorses that compete in the USA at the classic distances (2 to 2.4 km) do not need as many fast twitch, highly glycolytic fibers. These types of muscle fibers are critical for sprinters (Wood *et al.*, 1988) and would typically accompany a wider chest, but are less critical for many Thoroughbred racehorses that race at the longer distances (Mostert and Householder, 2000). Likewise, gaskin and forearm size are indicative of the composition of fast twitch and slow twitch fibers that the muscling contains. Typically, in terms of muscle size, one should be most concerned about the muscling over the horse's topline, including the back, the loin, and the croup, as that is where a horse generates its power. As is the case with halter horses, a horse should be wider at the stifle than across the top of the croup.

An absolute necessity for speed are short cannon bones, both front and back. The hocks and knees should be as low to the ground as possible. The pasterns should not be too short, nor should they be too long. Pasterns that are too short and upright limit stride length and cushion, but too-long pasterns also increase the likelihood of developing injuries (Barr, 1994). A horse that is a little upright in the pastern would probably be more desirable than a horse that is too long, especially if the horse had a long sloping shoulder that could absorb some of the additional shock that accompanies an upright pastern. The withers need to sit further back to allow for a longer, more sloping shoulder and, hence, a longer stride. The straighter the shoulder is, the shorter the stride. Very few champion horses have a short, upright shoulder.

A horse that is back-at-the-knees should be avoided. When running at speed, the carpus already tends to hyperextend. If the horse is back at its knees, this hyperextension is excessive and often results in carpal chips or fractures. Being slightly over-at-the-knee does not seem to be a major issue. However, research suggests carpal conformation can change between the time that a horse is a weanling and the time that is a three-year-old (McIlwraith *et al.*, 2003). A foal that is back-at-the-knee may improve though one that is over-at-the-knee may worsen. Additionally, being mildly offset at the knees, while not desirable, is not nearly as problematic as being back-at-the-knees. Likewise, a horse that turns out or turns in a little is not an issue as long as the horse moves well. When watching the horse move, it is critical to look for unusual joint movement, as this often translates into injuries. Curby-hocked or sickle-hocked horses are undesirable as it seems to take away from some of their power and may contribute to injuries (McIlwraith *et al.*, 2003).

The feet of a Thoroughbred racehorse undergo a tremendous amount of force while running, and horses with bad feet should be avoided. Mule-footed horses, which have narrow, oval feet with steep walls, are prone to injury, as are horses with dished-hooves. Having a 'platter-foot', or a very wide, flat hoof, on a racehorse is also undesirable. Given that the foot comes to a stop and then must accelerate at a high velocity, and repeat this as often as two and a half times per second when racing, any extra weight associated with the hoof requires extra energy. Hence, there is a compromise between having a foot that is large enough to support the horse but small enough to avoid wasted energy. It has been suggested that 'an ounce on the foot is like a pound on the back' (Ainslie, 1986). The accuracy of this statement remains to be determined, but unnecessarily large feet are disadvantageous.

Overall size of a horse does not matter as long as it is fast. A big horse takes fewer cycles or strides than a smaller horse to cover the same distance, but there have been many small horses that have been quite successful. These horses either had long strides despite their size, or took strides with greater frequency. For individuals interested in pursuing the classic distances, the trend is to select bigger, scopier-looking horses despite some recent examples in the United States of some relatively small horses winning the Kentucky Derby, including Mine That Bird and Smarty Jones.

Besides selecting horses to personally race, horses are sometimes purchased with the intention of 'pinhooking' them – or reselling them the following year without racing them prior to sale. Pinhooking can imply buying a weanling and selling it as a yearling, or it can mean purchasing a yearling in the fall, starting it under saddle, proceeding with race training, and then selling it as a two-year-old in training come spring. While most of the desirable qualities in a prospect will remain the same regardless of its final destination, there are a few traits that should be weighted differently depending upon what one plans to do with the horse.

When reselling a horse, it is helpful if the animal is of larger stature, with a refined head. A horse with a wide head and big eyes set out at the corners of the head (as opposed to a 'pig-eyed' horse) will have a greater field of vision and is not as easily startled. Additionally, it helps to create a more attractive animal and it is important to remember that 'pretty will always sell'. While 'no horse is ugly in the winner's circle', that is not the case in the sale ring. Thus, if the plan is to resell the horse, having a pretty horse will aid in getting that done.

While good conformation is important whether selecting a horse to resell or to race, the pedigree of a horse tends to dictate what will be the final purchase price. There are stallions capable of producing quality offspring that are not being marketed in the best fashion. They are not getting bred to the best mares and the offspring are not being put in position to be successful. As a result, the offspring from these stallions will often sell for less than the offspring from a stallion that is being managed in a way that will preserve the stallion's value by refusing to breed lower quality mares. If one is planning to personally race a horse, it is reasonable to consider offspring from stallions who have not been marketed as strategically, as you can often have success at a much lower cost. However, with pinhooking, there are advantages to working with the offspring of stallions that are being more properly marketed. Those horses will typically appear better in a sale's catalog as care will have been taken to ensure the stallion's statistics on his offspring are as good as possible.

It is often recommended that one should 'breed speed to speed' and 'type to type'. While it is true that such an approach results in many successful runners, it may be contributing to unsoundness issues. Considering that one of the consequences of breeding true to type is an increase in conformation problems, it is not surprising that racehorses experience a remarkably large amount of injuries. However, to win the shorter-distance races common in the United States, breeding horses specifically for speed makes sense and this trend will likely continue.

Most individuals recognize the importance of evaluating conformation, structure, and pedigree when selecting horses. However, the mentality of a horse can play a huge role in whether it will be successful. If one could measure the proverbial 'heart' of a horse, it would be possible to remove many prospects from your selection list. Unfortunately, that is not possible, but other parts of the horse's mental state can be evaluated. For instance, it is constructive to visit the barns when they are mostly deserted. During sales, there is a tremendous amount of commotion going on that may alter a horse's normal behavior. However, during off-times, it will be more obvious as to which horses walk their stalls, weave, kick the walls, or act nervous. It is also a good idea to ask the horse's handlers if the horse has been eating well at the sale. If a horse is not eating well at sales, it will probably not eat well when it is at the racetrack. A horse needs to eat wherever it is taken and avoiding a finicky eater can be useful.

In terms of temperament, numerous people consider Thoroughbred racehorses to be high-strung and somewhat uncontrollable. While there are certainly examples of such horses that were difficult to control and yet were successful on the track, there are many more horses that are much calmer and easier to handle. Nervous horses often fail to perform at their best (Cator, 1991), whereas calm horses more readily accept new situations. Race day can be quite stressful and it is the calm horse that will be better able to focus on racing and this increases the likelihood of reaching the winners' circle. Throughout the selection process, that is the ultimate goal.

References

Ainslie, T. (1986) Ainslie's Complete Guide to Thoroughbred Racing. 3rd ed. Simon & Schuster, New York.

Barr, A.R.S. (1994) Carpal conformation in relation to carpal chip fracture. Vet Rec 134, 646-650.

Brakenhoff, J.E., Holcombe, S.J., Hauptman, J.G., Smith, H.K., Nickels, F.A., Caron, J.P. (2006) The prevalence of laryngeal disease in a large population of competition draft horses. Vet Surg 35, 579-583.

Cator, R. (1991) Performance evaluations of racing Thoroughbreds. J Eq Vet Sci 11, 183-190.

Cook, W.R. (1988) Diagnosis and grading of hereditary recurrent laryngeal neuropathy in the horse. J Eq Vet Sci 8, 432-455.

Delahunty, D., Webb, S., Kelly, E.P., Smit, F.H. (1991) Intermandibular width and cannon bone length in 'winners' versus 'others'. J Eq Vet Sci 11, 258-259.

Jones, W.E. (1993) Left laryngeal hemiplegia. J Eq Vet Sci 13, 316-317.

McIlwraith, C.W., Anderson, T.M., Sanschi, E.M. (2003) Conformation and musculoskeletal problems in the racehorse. Clin Tech Equine Pract 2, 339-347.

Mostert, P.S., Householder, D.D. (2000) Intermandibular width as a selection criterion for Thoroughbreds. J Eq Vet Sci 20, 418-461.

Smith, A.M., Staniar, W.B., Splan, R.K. (2006) Associations between yearling body measurements and career racing performance in Thoroughbred racehorses. J Eq Vet Sci 26, 212-214.

Wood, C.H., Ross, T.T., Armstrong, J.B., Hall, D.C. (1988) Variations in muscle fiber composition between successfully and unsuccessfully raced Quarter Horses. J Eq Vet Sci 8, 217-220.

The high level Endurance horse

Endurance riding has been practiced historically for as long as the horse has been domesticated. Its origin lies in mans need travel as quick as possible from A to B. Since 1955 endurance riding has been a significant sporting activity and the Tevis Cup (from Lake Tahoe in Nevada to Auburn in California) is probably the first formal 160 km ride ever held. In Europe endurance competitions started in the 1960's. The FEI accepted endurance riding as an FEI equestrian discipline in 1982. The first European Championships over 160 km were organised in Florac in 1984 and the first World Championships in Rome in 1986.

Nowadays many people enjoy endurance riding at a variety of distance and speeds varying from a 40 km pleasure ride with 10 km/hour to a highly competitive 160 km endurance race with an average speed of 17 km/h over terrains with large changes in altitude and difficult footing up to 24 km/hour or even more in a flat race in desert conditions.

Over the last 5-10 years the differences between rides have been more clear. In the 'older' rides such as the Tevis Cup and 'Les 160 km de Florac' terrain difficulties (steep hills, difficult footing) require experienced horses and horsemanship. In the 'newer' rides, introduced by the Arabian countries the track is quite flat and sandy without any difficult hazards, although of course the desert is a significant hazard in its own right. The average speed on the 'tough terrain rides' is much lower than on the 'desert rides'.

Basically, every fit horse or pony is capable of finishing a shorter distance ride. However longer and faster rides add significantly to the demands. A good endurance horses needs two major attributes:

- mental endurance;
- physical fitness and ability.

Although physical capacities could be considered to be more important than mental capacities, the reverse is probably true. Endurance riding is not possible on a horse that does not actually enjoy the sport as it is impossible to force a horse to walk or run for 40 or more kilometres without unacceptable force. Additionally spurs and whips are not allowed in endurance competitions. There is, however, much more to be considered.

Mental demands

Important mental demands on endurance horses include:

- willingness to perform;
- willingness to eat, drink, rest, urinate and defecate during a ride;
- amenable temperament (although some very unpleasant horses perform well too);
- tolerance of transport and an ability to accept unfamiliar housing and management;
- a determined, alert, self-confident and active attitude during the ride.

A good endurance horse is well behaved and will remain in the speed (walk, trot or canter) until encouraged to do something else. During the ride the horse will take every opportunity to drink or eat. Some horses do this naturally and these have a big advantage in endurance riding. The same applies to urinating and defecating. A horse that does not want to do these natural necessities during a ride is not suitable for the sport as it is impossible to perform for 6-12 hours without urinating and/or defecating. A horse that takes every opportunity to rest and relax during pauses in competition (e.g. the vet gates) also has a significant advantage over a horse that does not have this ability.

Horses with an amenable temperament are easier and better to look after than a horse with an unpleasant character that bites and/or kicks. Fortunately most endurance horses are easy to handle and enjoy being 'pampered'.

A horse that travel easily and feels as comfortable in a strange environment as at home also has a big advantage; it will rest better and will be in a better physical and psychological condition at the start of a competition. A horse that is quiet during the start of a ride will conserve energy in the first phase by not 'fighting' its rider. Alertness for footing and 'self confidence' makes the ride more comfortable for horse and rider, and both will conserve energy.

Finally, horses that are able to relax quickly in a vet gate are more likely to pass the vet check shortly after arrival and therefore have a significant time advantage.

Physical attributes

Important physical attributes include:

- suitable conformation;
- good general health;
- soundness;
- comfortable gaits;
- strong feet;
- healthy tendons.

Although every healthy horse is able to perform an endurance ride, to be a winner over longer distances has obvious extra demands. When endurance competitions started in Europe some rather unexpected breeds, such as Warmbloods, Fjord horses and Icelandic horses, completed FEI 160 km rides. However, in those early days the maxim was 'to finish is to win'. Nowadays, the average speed of endurance rides has increased significantly and almost all participating horses are Arabians or Arabian crosses. Perhaps endurance 'races' is now a better reflection on the sport than endurance 'rides'.

Arabians are considered to be the most suitable breed as these have been bred for stamina and endurance. In general larger, heavier framed horses are less able to sustain the speeds required to win. Arabian horses have a very high percentage of type I oxidative fibres and a particular ability to utilise lipid energy sources during submaximal exercise, which makes this breed very suitable for endurance sport.

Suitable conformation is also important; small abnormalities in conformation can become significant handicaps on longer rides. Horses with obvious conformational defects will seldom manage to compete over the usual 4-10 year performance span and are therefore naturally excluded.

Horses that are required to perform for many hours need to have good general health. Even a minor gastrointestinal problem or a slight cough may become a serious issue after 140 km. A low resting heart rate and a very quick return to normal heart rate after exercise are a big advantage. Panting, quick superficial breathing, may also be advantageous in endurance horses as these horses are able to lose heat more quickly. A thin skin with good cutaneous circulation is also advantageous because body heat is an important issue in most rides. Horses with a thin well vascularised skin are easier to cool down during the ride.

Comfortable gaits are important to both rider and horse. The smoother the gait the more efficient and the less tiring for the rider. A non-tired rider stays better in balance and that's better for the gaits. Any movement away from the axis of a limb during the swing phase of the stride is a 'weakness' and this may become a problem after a longer distance. 'Interference' is a common problem in endurance horses and if the horse has a 'sway' action this is more likely to occur. Good hoof balance is also important in preventing interference. Strong 'clean' legs and feet without any disease or injury history are necessary to perform successfully in endurance. The tendons of endurance horses need to be 'clean' and free from previous injury as the demands are huge; even small alterations can turn into performance limiting damage over the course of training and competition.

Suspensory desmitis is the most common cause of lameness in endurance horses and frequently leads to termination of an endurance career. Superficial digital flexor tendonitis may be a problem in endurance horses like in all sport horses. Thorough ultrasonographic examination of all the major limb tendons is important in endurance horses; the slightest lesions can lead to long layoffs.

Foot problems are also significant performance limiting factors. Bruising during a ride and laminitis are probably the best examples of the type of injuries that cause problems. Laminitis can arise from direct trauma through long distances on hard surfaces ('road founder'), and may also be a result of serious metabolic disturbances; both may occur in endurance riding. A horse with a history of laminitis is more likely to experience recurrence, and thus horses with a history of laminitis are less suitable for endurance sport.

Myositis is also a constant threat to the endurance horse. Coupled with metabolic abnormalities this can be life-threatening.

Last but not least: if the rider becomes fatigued during a ride paravertebral myalgia of the horse may become a problem as the rider is not in balance anymore. Sufficient riding experience and the physical fitness of the rider are very important in endurance riding. A ride strategy based on the known abilities of the horse and the specific demands of the course (elevation, footing etc.) are important aspects of successful endurance performance.

Conclusion

A good modern endurance horse is often an Arab or an Arab-cross with optimal conformation, a flexible character and above all 'a will to win'. It is the task of the ride veterinarians to keep the 'will to win' of horse and rider within limits to protect the health and welfare of the competing horses.

References

Bergero, D., Assenza, A., Caola, G. (2005) Contribution to our knowledge of the physiology and metabolism of endurance horses. Livestock Production Sci 92, 167-176.

Foss, M.A., Wickler, S.J. (2004) Veterinary aspects of endurance riding. In: Hinchcliff, K.W., Kaneps, A.J., Geor, R.J. (eds.) Equine sports medicine and surgery. Saunders, Elsevier Limited. Pp 1105-1117.

Misheff, M.M. (2003) Lameness in endurance horses. In: Ross, M.W., Dyson, S.J. (eds.) Lameness in the horse. Saunders, Elsevier Science, St. Louis. p 996-1002.

Ricard, A., Touvais, M. (2007) Genetic parameters of performance traits in horse endurance races. Livestock Sci 110, 118-125.

Sloet van Oldruitenborgh-Oosterbaan, M.M., Wensing, Th., Barneveld, A., Breukink, H.J. (1991) Heart rate, blood biochemistry and performance in horses, competing in a 100 km endurance ride. Vet Rec 128, 175-179.

Sloet van Oldruitenborgh-Oosterbaan, M.M. (2004) Does heart rate indicate the health status of endurance horses during competition? Conference on Equine Sports Medicine and Science, Oslo, September 23-25, 2004. In: Lindner, A. (ed.) The elite race and endurance horse. Lensing Druck, Dortmund, Germany. p. 91-97.

Sloet van Oldruitenborgh-Oosterbaan, M.M. (2005) Problems facing the endurance horse. In: Proc British Equine Vet Assoc Annual Congress, Harrogate, UK. p 75-77.

Performance evaluation for the prepurchase examination: How it is done in the Netherlands

M.M. Sloet van Oldruitenborgh-Oosterbaan
Department of Equine Sciences, Faculty of Veterinary Medicine, Utrecht University, Yalelaan 114, 3584 CM Utrecht, the Netherlands

Introduction

Dutch horses have a high reputation and are sold worldwide, therefore the protocols used by Dutch veterinarians for pre-purchase examination need to be of an exemplary standard. In the Netherlands the pre-purchase examination (PPE) has been standardised since 1983 through the use of a handbook and a prescribed protocol (Wagenaar, 1983), both of which have been updated regularly with the latest version (2007) being widely accepted as the gold standard for the procedure (Sloet van Oldruitenborgh-Oosterbaan *et al.*, 2007).

Selection of a veterinarian

In contrast to some other countries, in the Netherlands both the vendor and the purchaser can select a veterinarian to perform the prepurchase examination. As a result horses may be examined on behalf of the vendor or on behalf of the prospective purchaser. The general advice is always that the client (vendor or purchaser) chooses a veterinarian he likes and trusts. However, since 2000 an official registry of 'certified prepurchase examination veterinarians' has been developed. In March 2010, 47 equine veterinarians were registered. In order to qualify for registration veterinarians must have successfully completed an evaluation of their clinical skills (mainly centred on the quality and correct interpretation of radiographs) and an inspection of their facilities. The latter includes a soft-surface lunging area, a hard surface track and a hard surface lunging circle. The evaluation of the facilities and the subsequent random checking of completed pre-purchase examinations (including complete sets of radiographs) are undertaken by an independent, certified, quality control organisation, aided by a group of veterinary experts. The overall organisation and registration is supervised by an independent group 'Stichting Paard', that consists of 'stake holders' in the equine industry such as insurance companies, breed associations and dealers. Certified PPE-veterinarians are obliged to attend specific CPD courses and general equine CPD. The advice provided by the certified PPE veterinarian will be accepted by the insurance companies without further examination.

The introduction of the 'certified PPE vet' in the Netherlands significantly improved the quality of the examination and more or less guarantees objective information provision, thus enabling laymen and other parties involved to purchase horses with confidence. Conflicts of interest arising when a veterinarian who is directly involved with a particular horse, is asked to examine the same horse for a purchaser, are overcome by the seller agreeing that all relevant information can be divulged.

Performance evaluation during a prepurchase examination

Contrary to the approach in some other European countries, in the Netherlands the veterinarian who performs the prepurchase examination will not evaluate the performance of the horse. It is the responsibility of the prospective purchaser to evaluate retrospectively the sport performance of the horse by either checking the competition records of the Dutch National Equestrian Federation or by checking FEI data. Further, it is also the responsibility of the purchaser to evaluate the abilities of the horse for the intended purpose. On the form (See Appendix 1) only the 'level of training according to client' is noted. The veterinarian does not have a duty to check this in any manner.

During the clinical stage of the prepurchase exam the horse is lunged for 10-15 minutes on a soft surface at walk, trot and canter. During this examination the locomotion is assessed and particular attention is paid to any abnormal respiratory noises. Immediately after the lunging exercise the heart and lungs are auscultated on both sides for rhythm and abnormal sounds.

In the Netherlands during a standardized prepurchase examination the horse is not observed during its normal work (dressage, jumping, eventing, etc.). This is an approach that is widely accepted and although incidentally an individual veterinarian, especially if his client is the purchaser, may evaluate the horse also during riding or driving, this is not a standard requirement.

Prepurchase examination report

The official form as issued by the Royal Netherlands Veterinary Association (KNMvD), shown in Appendix 1. (original A3 format), is widely used by Dutch equine practitioners to report the results of PPE. These are uniquely numbered carbon copy forms: one for the client (often laminated to prevent unauthorised alterations) and one for the clinician to store in the archives (mandatory retention for 10 years). On these forms it is stated that: 'The prepurchase examination was performed using the handbook 'De veterinaire keuring van het paard' issue 2007 as guidance'.

The left-hand half of the form deals mainly with information concerning the client, the horse and the clinician performing the examination. Information on behavioural vices and blood samples is also included here. The client (vendor or purchaser) is required to sign the form before the examination starts to confirm that an agreement exists concerning the general conditions of the examination. At the end of the process the veterinarian will provide the conclusion of his findings and sign the form.

Clinical examination

On the right-hand side of the form the results of the clinical and radiological examinations are described. As mentioned previously the full examination is performed following the standard protocol and thus the description on the form can be brief.

Clinical examination consists of:
- a general physical and clinical examination;
- an inspection palpation and percussion of the head, rump and limbs;
- inspection and percussion of the hooves;
- inspection at the walk and trot on a hard surface and walk, trot and canter on a soft surface;
- the performance of flexion tests.

Radiographic examination

Most horses that are subjected to a prepurchase examination will also be examined radiographically. If the horse is to be insured for over € 4,500, a radiological assessment is mandatory.

On the right-hand side of the form the number of radiographs and the radiological report are entered. Based on the information gained by 20 standard views, further radiological investigations may be indicated.

The basic standard views used in the Netherlands are:
- LF and RF feet – Lateromedial and Dorso 55° Proximal-PalmaroDistal Oblique = upright pedal view, centred on the navicular bone (4 views).
- LF and RF fetlock – Lateromedial + Dorso 45° Lateral-PalmaroMedial Oblique and Dorso 45° Medial-PalmaroLateral Oblique (6 views).
- LH and RH tarsal (2 views).
- LH and RH fetlock joint - Lateromedial (2 views); where there are questionable findings additional oblique views are undertaken.
- LH and RH stifle joint – Lateromedial; if suspicious changes are identified additional plantaro-dorsal view and/or Caudal 10° Proximal 60° Latero-Cranio Medial Oblique views are obtained (2-6 views).

The interpretation of the radiographs is based on the grading system published by Dik KJ (Wagenaar, 1983; Sloet van Oldruitenborgh-Oosterbaan *et al.*, 2007): grade 1 being 'ideal' and grade 4 being 'poor'. All other radiographic detectable changes, not included in the grading system descriptions are described in full. The implications of the clinical interpretations may, however, vary between observers. Variations in interpretation can arise from the age and use of the horse and its intended purpose.

Joint fragments (osteochondrosis, chip fragments etc.) frequently give rise to discussion when considering the clinical relevance and risk assessment. For this reason the major Dutch insurance company Hippo Zorg BV, in dialogue with experienced senior equine clinicians, have developed a transparent scheme for the evaluation of osteochondrotic lesions and fragmentation of the fetlock, the tarsal and the stifle joints. This scheme is now the accepted standard in the Netherlands (Sloet van Oldruitenborgh-Oosterbaan *et al.*, 2007).

The standard clinical and radiological protocols should only be considered to be a starting point. Additional diagnostic procedures such as ultrasound or endoscopy can be performed if indicated or if specifically requested by the purchaser. The results of any extra examinations are described under 'other remarks'.

Conclusion

Performance evaluation for a prepurchase examination is not the standard in the Netherlands. The inventory of a horse is suitable for the intended purchaser (rider or driver) and for the intended sport discipline is completely the responsibility of the purchaser. The veterinarian who performs the prepurchase examination will record all abnormal findings and provide a qualified opinion and a risk assessment based on up-to-date veterinary knowledge. The conclusion of the examination is not a declaration as to whether the horse is suitable for a particular rider or a specific future athletic use.

The copy of the form, the radiographs in hard copy or digital format and all other relevant information should be retained by the examining veterinarian for 10 years.

References

Wagenaar, G.J. (1983). De keuring van het paard. Wetenschappelijke Uitgeverij Bunge.

Sloet van Oldruitenborgh-Oosterbaan, M.M., Barneveld, A., Van den Belt, A.J. (2007) De veterinaire keuring van het paard. Uitgeverij Libre B.V. Leeuwarden, the Netherlands.

Appendix 1.

Clinical examination report

Number:

(Formulated by the Netherlands Equine Veterinary Association of the Royal Netherlands Veterinary Association.
The pre-purchase examination was performed using the handbook "De veterinaire keuring van het paard" issue 2007 as a guidance).

Client: ______

Address: ______

Zip code / City: ______

Client is present at the exam: yes / no

Client is: buyer / seller / other, namely ______

Level of training (according to client): ______

Proposed use (according to client): breeding / sport

Location where the exam takes place: clinic / other, namely ______

Signalment:

Name: ______

Breed or type: ______

Studbook no.: ______

Microchip number: ______

Pedigree: ______

Age: ______ Sex: ______

Coat colour: ______ Height at withers +/- ______

Markings:

Head: ______

LF: ______ LH: ______

RF: ______ RH: ______

Other: ______

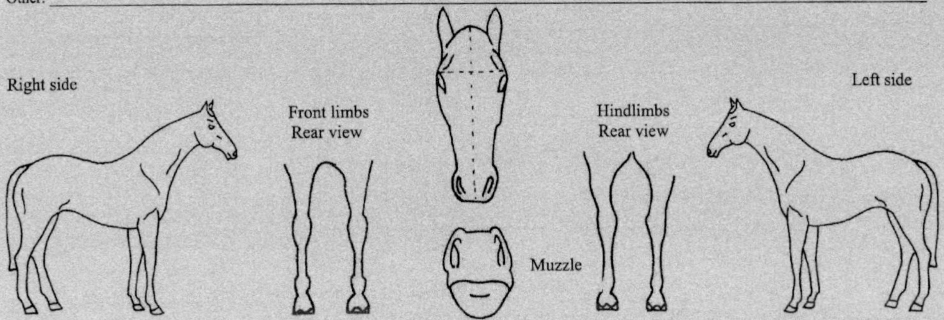

Evidence seen of possible behavioural vices? yes / none (If yes; Details ....)
Blood collected and put into custody by the examining veterinary surgeon? yes / no
Blood sample tested for prohibited substances at client's request ? yes / no

Veterinary practice (stamp):

1. The examining veterinary surgeon and/or veterinary practice shall not be held liable for loss or damage caused as a result of the performance of the examination or as a result of inaccuracies or shortcomings in their preparation of this report, unless it has been established that this loss or damage is due to malice or negligence on the part of the examining veterinary surgeon.
2. The client shall have the sole right to invoke any action due to liability on the part of the examining veterinary surgeon and/or veterinary practice as described under 1 above. Parties other than the client shall not be entitled to derive any rights to compensation for damages arising from this examination/report.
3. Liability shall be limited at all times to that amount covered by the veterinary surgeon's professional indemnity insurance applicable at the time of the examination. Details of this coverage in the form of policy documents for this insurance may be inspected at the veterinary practice premises, and copies of these may be obtained at first request from the veterinary practice at no charge.
4. The provisions printed on this examination report shall also apply in the event the client fails to sign this form, or refuse to accept receipt of this examination report.
5. If the client upon whose instructions the examination was performed is not the owner of the horse, the client is wholly responsible for having obtained the owner's consent to all procedures performed during the examination, and the client shall fully indemnify the veterinary surgeon in respect of any claim by the owner arising from an allegation that such consent was not given.
6. In the event the client and/or third parties are of the opinion that the health of the horse at the time of the present examination does not correspond to that which is stated in the examination report, these parties must report this to the other party without delay and in writing (for example, together with the purchase contract), under penalty of the lapsing of every right of action against the examining veterinarian and/or the veterinarian practice, and to hold this party liable for compensation, while also simultaneously providing a copy of this report to the examination veterinarian and the veterinarian practice.
7. The laws of the Netherlands shall apply exclusively to any disputes arising from the performance of the examination and/or the completion of the examination report, and the Court of the Netherlands shall retain sole jurisdiction to hear these disputes.
8. In the event of differing interpretations between the Dutch and English text of these conditions, the content of the Dutch text shall be decisive.

Signature of Client:

______

CONCLUSION: ______

Thus examined and reported by me:

______

veterinary surgeon in:

______

This report can relate only to the appearance on the date of examination ....

Signature of examining veterinary surgeon:

______

Clinical examination report

Number:

General and clinical examination:

	normal	abnormal	
conformation and stance	☐	☐	______
condition	☐	☐	______
skin and coat	☐	☐	______
mucous membranes	☐	☐	______
lymph nodes	☐	☐	______
eyes and eyelids	☐	☐	______
Respiratory system			
respiration at rest	☐	☐	______
type of respiration	☐	☐	______
spontaneous coughing	no	yes	______
larynx sensitivity	☐	☐	______
respiration after exercise	☐	☐	______
abnormal sounds	no	yes	______
laryngoscopy performed	no	yes	______
laryngoscopy findings	☐	☐	______
Circulatory system			
peripheral circulation	☐	☐	______
heart at rest	☐	☐	______
heart after exercise	☐	☐	______
Digest. system (ext. insp.)	☐	☐	______
mouth, teeth, tongue	☐	☐	______
Urogen. system (ext. insp.)	☐	☐	______
Nervous system			
tail tone	☐	☐	______
correction reflexes	☐	☐	______
coordination	☐	☐	______

Inspection, palpation and eventual percussion:

	normal	abnormal	
head	☐	☐	______
neck	☐	☐	______
withers	☐	☐	______
back	☐	☐	______
croup	☐	☐	______
left frontlimb	☐	☐	______
right frontlimb	☐	☐	______
left hindlimb	☐	☐	______
right hindlimb	☐	☐	______
Hooves			
horn quality	☐	☐	______
hoof percussion	☐	☐	______
hoof shape	even / uneven	…… higher than …..	
shoeing	no / front / front and hind		
type of shoeing	______		

Walk, trot and canter:

	normal	abnormal	
Walking on hard surface			
straight line	☐	☐	______
small circle on the left	☐	☐	______
small circle on the right	☐	☐	______
Trotting on hard surface			
straight line	☐	☐	______
small circle on the left	☐	☐	______
small circle on the right	☐	☐	______
Trotting on soft surface			
small circle on the left	☐	☐	______
small circle on the right	☐	☐	______
Cantering on soft surface			
small circle on the left	☐	☐	______
small circle on the right	☐	☐	______

Flexion tests:

Forced flexion: Trotting after 1 min. flexion:

	-	±	+	++
LF not sensitive / sensitive	LF ☐	☐	☐	☐
RF not sensitive / sensitive	RF ☐	☐	☐	☐
LH not sensitive / sensitive	LH ☐	☐	☐	☐
RH not sensitive / sensitive	RH ☐	☐	☐	☐

Radiological examination performed: ☐ yes ☐ no

Number of X-rays ______

Assessment of radiographs:

Grading

Navicular bone	LF		RF	
Fetlock joint	LF		RF	
Sesamoid bones	LF		RF	
Tarsal joint	LH		RH	

		Fragments -	+	**Remarks**
Fetlock joint	LF	☐	☐	______
Fetlock joint	RF	☐	☐	______
Stifle joint	LH	☐	☐	______
Stifle joint	RH	☐	☐	______
Tarsal joint	LH	☐	☐	______
Tarsal joint	RH	☐	☐	______
Fetlock joint	LH	☐	☐	______
Fetlock joint	RH	☐	☐	______

Radiological exam of other parts / extra findings:

______

______

______

______

______

______

Other remarks:

______

______

______

______

______

______

______

Performance evaluation for training guidance

Anne Couroucé-Malblanc[1]*, Gustaf Croon*[2]*, Arne Lindholm*[2]*, Arno Lindner*[3] *and Björn Nolting*[4]

[1]*Pathologie Médicale des Equidés, Unité de Médecine, Ecole Nationale Vétérinaire, Atlanpole - La Chantrerie BP 40706, 44307 Nantes cedex 03, France*

[2]*Mälaren Equine clinic, Hälgesta 1, 19391 Sigtuna, Sweden*

[3]*Heinrich-Röttgen-Str. 20, 52428 Jülich, Germany*

[4]*Tierärztliche Praxis für Pferde, Dr. Björn Nolting GmbH, Heimerzheimer Str. 18, 53919 Weilerswist, Germany*

Introduction

Performance evaluation or diagnostics permits identification of horses that are best trained and more capable of performing in sports and to assess the effectiveness of training programs. In some instances the methods used for performance diagnostics allow for guiding the training of horses also. This article presents the approaches of several authors to provide this service.

For performance diagnostics horses can be submitted to standardized exercise tests to determine their individual blood [LA]-running speed (BLRS) and heart rate-running speed (HRRS) relationships. The BLRS curves and HRRS lines themselves can be used to compare horses, but more frequently, their parameters are derived for use as performance diagnostics. The most often derived parameter of the BLRS relationship is the v_4 (velocity run under defined conditions inducing a blood [LA] of 4 mmol/L; Persson, 1983; Lindner, 2000). The v_{200} is frequently calculated as the parameter representing the HRRS (velocity run under defined conditions inducing a heart rate of 200 beats/min; Persson, 1983; Couroucé, 1997).

Approach Couroucé-Malblanc

Method

Realization of standardized exercise tests is important to define the exercise ability of three-day-event horses. Some studies have previously described exercise test protocols for three-day-event horses (Auvinet *et al.*, 1989; Galloux, 1991; Hasson, 1994; Munoz *et al.*, 1998; Van Erck, 2005). Various key points of these standardized exercise tests will be discussed thereafter according to these studies and to the author practical experience:

1. Number of steps. Three steps seem sufficient to measure the regression line between heart rate (HR) and velocity (V) and the exponential curve for blood

lactate concentration vs velocity. A fourth step may be added if needed but more than 4 steps seem not realizable for practical reasons.

2. Duration of each step. The duration of each step should be sufficient to reach a steady state for blood lactate concentration and heart rate. According to Munoz *et al.* (1998), a constant HR seems to be reached after 40 sec of exercise. For blood lactate concentration, the minimal duration is not precisely defined. However, a step duration of 2 min 30 sec to 3 min as recommended by Auvinet *et al.* (1989) and Galloux *et al.* (1991) may be a good compromise between physiological and practical requirements.
3. Recovery between the steps. The recovery period between each step maybe of about 2 min in order to have no cumulative effect for blood lactate concentration.
4. Intensity of each step. In a study performed by van Erck *et al.* (2005), 10 healthy three-day-event horses performed a standardized exercise test on a race track with 4 steps each of 1000 m. For each step, velocity was increased up to maximal velocity on the 4th step. For these horses, a 4 mmol/l blood lactate concentration was reached for a mean velocity of 30.7 ± 1.2 km/h (512 ± 20 m/min) and a HR of 174 ± 9 bpm. This study shows that V_{170} is closely related to V_4 in three-day-event horses which is also highly correlated to performance (Leleu *et al.*, 2005).

Therefore, in my opinion to have standardized exercise test protocols with submaximal exercise adapted to all horses, three-day event horses may be submitted to 3 steps of 3 min each, the aim being to reach a HR >170 bpm and a blood lactate concentration >4 mmol/l at the end of the third step.

As tracks on which three-day-events horses exercise are very different (grass or sand race-tracks grass, sand training tracks, sand on the beach, ...) it is often difficult to define the intensity of the steps by giving a velocity to the rider. It may also be difficult for an unexperienced rider to gallop horses at defined heart rates and to maintain constant speeds of exercise according to the recommendations. Therefore, in practice, it is often useful to define the intensity according to the gallop of the horse: moderate gallop, medium gallop, fast gallop. As the rider knows both the horse and the track, it usually leads to an exercise with each step being at constant intensity and with an increasing intensity from one step to the other.

Guiding

The three-day-event horse is a 'complete athlete' and needs to perform well in dressage, cross-country and show jumping. Therefore, two different kinds of exercises are needed during training:

1. Technical exercises to develop dressage and jumping abilities with lunge work, dressage, jumping (work over obstacles), jumping (gymnastics).
2. Exercises to improve the aerobic capacity of the horse and it's ability to tolerate high blood lactate concentration.

Three-day-event horses should reach blood lactate concentration between 2 and 4 mmol/l during training in order to do real aerobic capacity work (Courouçé, 1998, 1999; Leleu *et al.*, 2005). This kind of work may be included in endurance or canter exercises as steps of 2 to 3 min at an intensity between HR_2 and HR_4, which means mainly between 160 and 170 bpm. These exercises may help to increase the horse's aerobic capacity and thus delay blood lactate accumulation (Courouçé, 1998). These exercises may be performed once or twice a week, during 4 to 6 weeks and maybe done between two competitions if the period between them is above 3 weeks.

Also, as horses reach blood lactate concentration between 10 and 20 mmol/l after the cross, it is particularly important to prepare the horse to accumulate and tolerate such lactate concentrations in the muscles and in the blood. To accomplish this the exercise should be of high intensity and short duration. This means canter with phases of 30 sec to 1 min with HR above HR4, which means above 170 bpm. Number of workouts needs to be adapted to each horse and each track. However, before realizing such exercises, it is important that horses develop their aerobic capacity with exercises such as previously described. These exercises should be done no more than once a week with a 10 days recovery period between the exercise and the competition.

Approach Lindholm and Croon

Blood lactate and heart rate measurements for performance evaluation and training guidance of the individual horse, in Standardbred and Coldblooded trotters, are not regularly used in Sweden. Most trainers use a private training camp. These camps are all very different and the training regimes differ between trainers. Straight tracks of various lengths (400-1,500 meters) are commonly used for interval training. Thousand meters oval tracks (race type track) are used for heat training and road-tracks are used for low intensity trotting. Only a few of the trainers use objective values of the intensity in their training regimes. The majority only use velocity as indicator of the training intensity.

Method

In order to assess the effectiveness and intensity of regular training programs performed at training camps we start by testing the daily training regimes. Detailed information about the training is obtained from the trainer to enable blood lactate measuring, with Lactate Pro, at strategic places. Heart rate, velocity and altitude are continually measured and recorded, with Polar S710 heart rate meter, during training.

After these initial tests of the (weekly) training, each horse performs a standardized exercise test (SET) on the 1000 meter race-track. The test starts with a 20 minutes jog (heart rate 140-180) and then a five minutes rest. The horse then performs four intervals of 1000 meters, each interval at a higher velocity then the one before. Constant velocity within each interval is desired but not easily obtained. The velocity in the first two intervals are based on age, sex and performance in the training regime test, aiming for blood lactate levels well under 4 mmol/l. The velocity in the third and fourth intervals are adjusted according to the result after the first and second intervals, aiming for blood lactate levels close to 10 mmol/l in the fourth interval. If the horse doesn´t reach desired blood lactate level in the fourth interval a fifth interval is conducted at even higher velocity. After each 1000 meter heat blood is immediately taken and blood lactate measured. The running times during intervals range from 90-130 seconds. The recovery period between each interval is three minutes. Heart rate is registered during the SET. VLa4 and V200 are calculated. After the last heat the horse is walked on the track for ten minutes and post exercise lactate is measured.

We also practice a SET, measuring and comparing heart rate during fixed conditions, same velocity and distance (Figure 1). This SET is easily performed by the trainers themselves and can be adjusted after almost any training facility.

Results

Figure 1 shows a test of the daily training regime. This is an initial test to obtain objective values of the intensity of the training that this horse is submitted to by his trainer.

Figure 2 shows the heart rate and velocity of a horse during a SET. Four intervals are performed at increasing velocity for each interval. The velocity differs slightly within the intervals, considered normal variation.

Figure 3 shows the result of the SET in Figure 2 (third test) and an earlier test (first test), comparing blood lactate at different velocities. The first test was performed five months earlier than the third test. A second test was performed between the first and the third test but is not shown in the figure. A significant improvement of the blood lactate – running speed curve is evident and therefore the VLa4 of the horse has increased substantially.

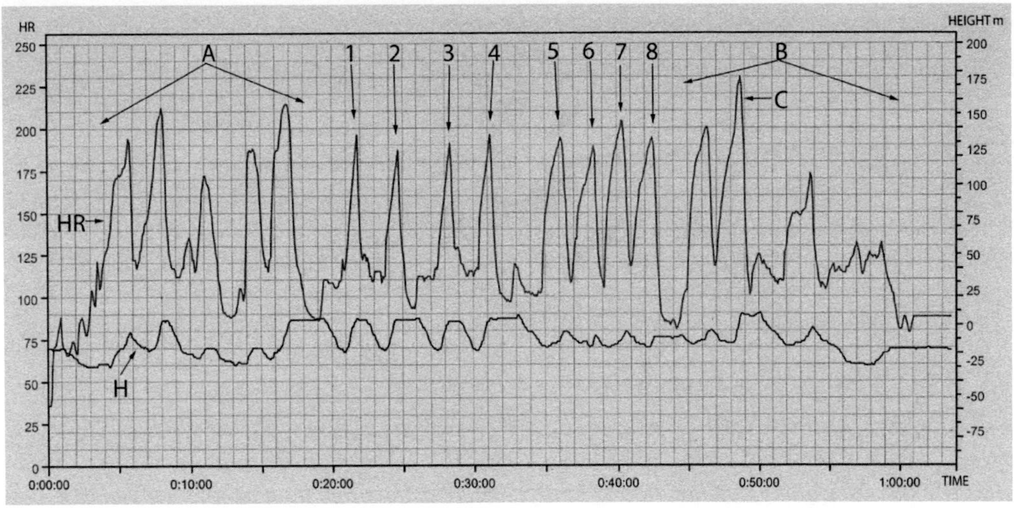

Figure 1. Coldblooded trotter, five year old stallion. Registration of heart rate (HR) and elevation covered (H) during a training session. The session starts with a tough 'warm up' (A) followed by four intervals (1-4) in short and steep hills. The training time in these hills is too short for sufficient aerobic training. Intervals 1-4 is about 30 seconds with a top HR of 190-195. Blood lactate was measured after interval 2 and 4, 2: 13.2 mmol/l lactate, 4: 15.1 mmol/l lactate, showing a high anaerobic demand. The training session continues with another four Intervals (5-8) on a straight track and ends with jog and walk (B). Ironically it´s in the jog that the horse reaches its highest HR (C).

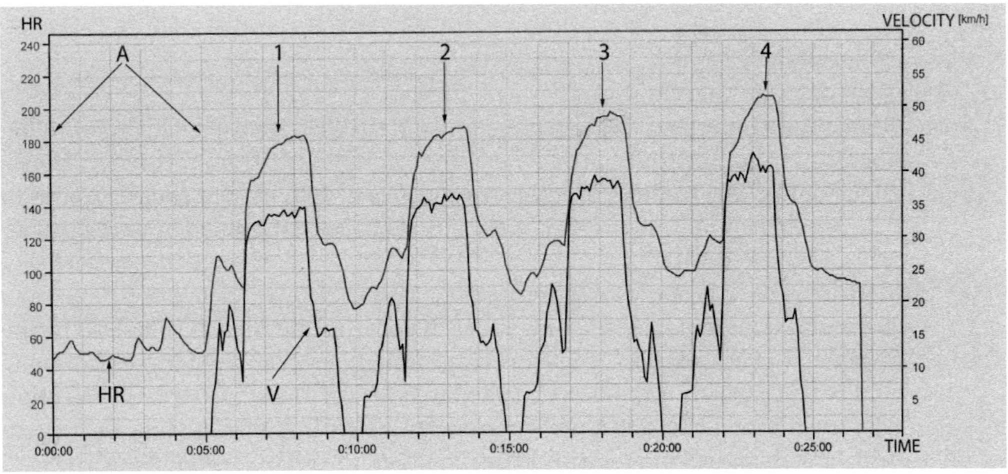

Figure 2. Coldblooded trotter, five year old stallion. Measuring heart rate (HR) and velocity (V) during standardized lactate test. The test starts with a warm up (not in the picture) and then a rest of five minutes (A). The horse then makes four intervals (1-4) on a race track of 1000 meters, each interval at a higher velocity. After each interval, blood lactate is measured: 1: 1.8 mmol/l lactate, 2: 2.9 mmol/l lactate, 3: 4.5 mmol/l lactate, 4: 8.3 mmol/l lactate.

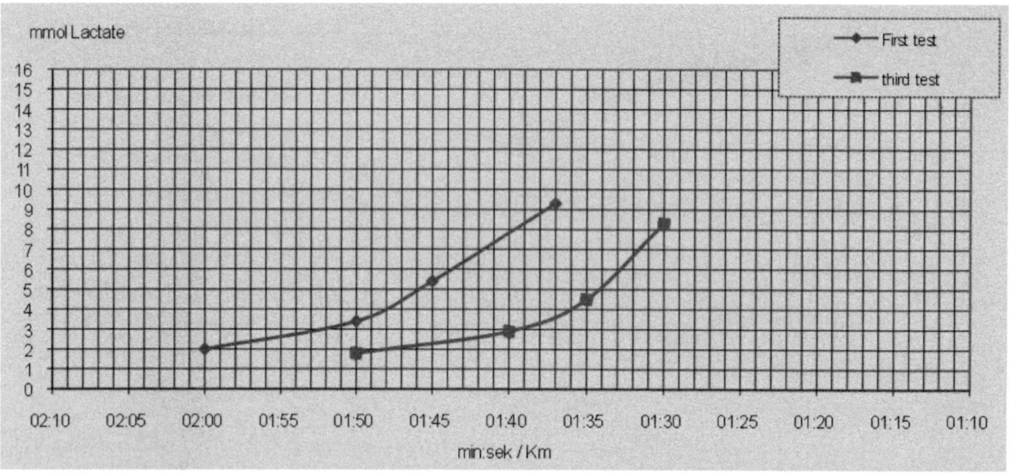

Figure 3. Blood lactate measured during standardized test, plotted against interval velocity. Two tests are shown, first test (rhombus) and third test (squares). Conditions are the same for both tests, which is required to enable performance evaluation. VLa4 is higher during the third test indicating an improvement in performance.

Figure 4 shows two SETs. Heart rate is measured during the tests which are conducted under the same conditions, velocity and distance. The heart rates from the two tests are compared. The HR is considerably lower in the second test than the first indicating an improvement in performance.

Discussion

The results from the training regime test and the SET are used when modifying the training regime, and guiding the trainer to individual training for each horse. Since only a few trainers use objective values of intensity in their training in Sweden there is no surprise that the training has been modified by every trainer we have worked with.

To be able to optimise the training for each horse, the performance test should be conducted every 8 weeks. This is a compromise between physiologic, economic and practical reasons that have worked well for us. This enables early detection of poor training effect and poor performance. With regular testing each horse will have a 'baseline' record making it easier to discover poor performance. Objective values of each horse's capability simplify the efforts of the trainers to create correct groups of horses that train together.

We have noticed a lower VLa4 in females compared to males in the same age group and on the same training schedule as the colts. Also noticed during

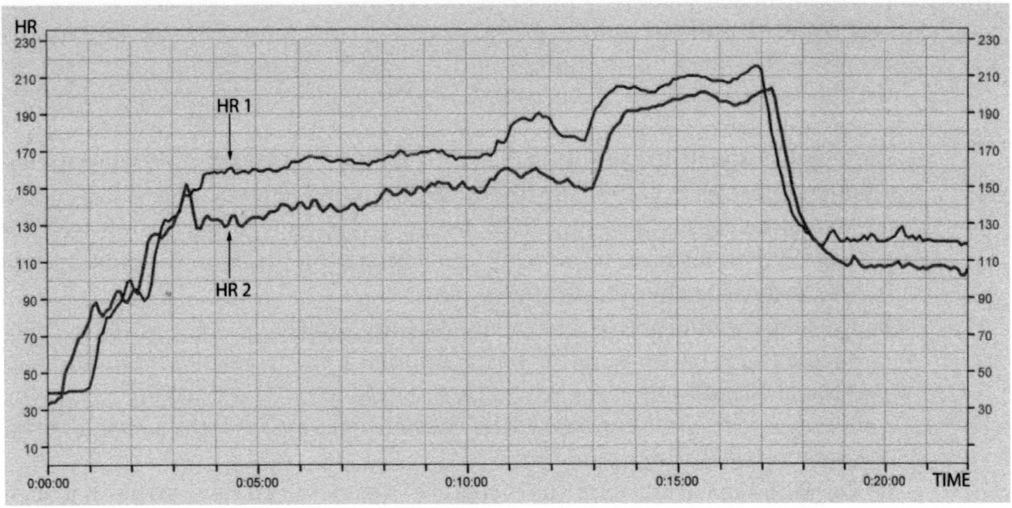

Figure 4. Standardbred trotter, six year old stallion. Standardized test measuring heart rate. Two tests are shown. The horse has undergone a regular training regime during 3 months between the tests. The conditions, velocity and distance are the same in both tests. Heart rate in the first test (HR1), heart rate in the second test (HR2). The HR is lower in the second test than the first test indicating an improvement in performance.

work with training guidance is the superior training effect achieved during the winter rather than the summer. This might be explained by the fact that most horses compete during summer at the cost of training sessions, suggesting that competition is not an optimal training. Both these observations have to be corroborated in a study in both breeds.

At the end of the SET the horse is walked on the track and post exercise lactate is measured. This gives a 'clearance value' for blood lactate. We believe that this value is less affected by surrounding factors such as track condition and weather because of the low velocity work. However, this also remains to be demonstrated.

Conclusions from practical training guidance:

1. The most common problem during training is the use of regimes of too high intensity leading eventually to injury. Too short a training time when short uphill trotting is performed, results in a high anaerobic demand without sufficient aerobic training.
2. Repeated performance evaluation with a standardized exercise test in the field is a good indicator of training effectiveness. Both V200- and VLa4-tests are easy to perform and widely accepted as indicators of training effectiveness.
3. All trainers taking part in our tests have modified their training regimes after receiving objective measurements of their training methods.

Approach Lindner

Method

The exercise speed to condition horses is defined by blood [LA] determined submitting horses to a SET. The SET prescription is (references in Table 1):

1. At least 4 steps (or intervals; steps are defined by time to be run, intervals are defined by a distance to be run) to obtain a blood [LA] of 4 mmol/l: three before and one after the 4 mmol/l value.
2. The steps at the speeds to be defined have a duration of 5 minutes each. The intervals have a duration of ≥ 5 minutes to allow the horses to finish an interval at the same place where they started and for not having to run the horses as fast as it is necessary with shorter steps. This is especially of interest when the tracks are not optimal.
3. The initial speed as well as the increase of speed in each step (interval) is such that at least 3 values of blood [LA] are obtained before the value of 4 mmol/l is reached or surpassed. This approach also allows to reduce the maximal speed needed to obtain a blood [LA] of ≥ 4 mmol/l.

Table 1. Studies published on conditioning horses with lactate guided speeds of exercise.

Author	Exercise					Horses		Effect
	Speed	Duration (minutes)	Frequency	Duration of conditioning period	SET	Breed (number)	Age (years)	on v_4 (%)
Werkmann *et al.*, 1996; Rivero *et al.*, 2006, 2007	$v_{2.5}$	5	Every 2nd day	3 weeks	Before and after	THB (6)	2-3	+ 1.6
	$v_{2.5}$	15		3 weeks				+ 2.5
	$v_{2.5}$	25		3 weeks				+ 4,1
	v_4	5		3 weeks				+ 3.7
	v_4	15		3 weeks				+ 2.1
	v_4	25		3 weeks				+ 4.8
Dag 1998; Gansen *et al.*, 1999; Lindner *et al.*, 2009	$v_{1.5}$	45	Every 2nd day	6 weeks	Before and after	Haflinger (6)	2	+ 7.3
	$v_{2.5}$	45		6 weeks				+ 4.9
	v_4	25		6 weeks				+ 2.3
Trilk *et al.*, 2002	v_2	45	Every 2nd day	6 weeks	Before and every 2 weeks	Diverse (6)	3-10	+ 17
Lindner *et al.*, 2007	v_{10}	2 x 5	Every 3rd day	6 weeks	Before and every 2 weeks	AA (5)	3-6	+ 14.1
Lindner *et al.*, 2010	v_{10}	2 x 5	Every 2nd day	6 weeks	Before and every 2 weeks	THB (6)	3-6	0

Results of guidance studies

In the initial studies, several different types of exercise were examined on the same horses (Werkman *et al.*, 1996; Gansen *et al.*, 1999), but later it was started to investigate the effect of onc type of exercise only, keeping the experimental conditions the same as much as possible in all experiments but for the type of exercise examined. Very many variables are measured on the horses during these experiments, but the one considered most important because of its practical value for performance diagnosis is v_4 (Lindner 2000, 2010). The aim in all studies is to increase the v_4 of the horses to give them a larger likelihood of performing well (Lindner 2000, 2010). The studies published so far are shown in Table 1.

Obviously studies on the effect of conditioning horses with exercise consisting of other combinations of duration, frequency, recovery time and blood lactate guided speeds will have to be performed. However, the effects of the blood lactate guided exercises shown in Table 1 already allow for an objective assessment of which ones are more effective. The practice will have to do the comparison between them and the conventionally used conditioning programs.

Approach Nolting

Training horses used for dressage

The word dressage is very often understood in a negative way. The meaning of the dressage training is not that the horses perform some movements in order to impress the judges or the naive audience. The dressage work of a horse is synonym for gymnastic work of the horse.

This is because the horse never was intended by nature as a mount. Although humans have bred the horse throughout history for their needs as a riding and driving horse, the horse`s back, because of its anatomy, is actually not designed to carry heavy loads.

Looking at the horse once from the side, it is striking that the main mass of the body, head, neck and chest is hung near the front. This weight is mainly carried by the front legs of the horse.

Now the extra weight of the rider is added to the back. Previously it was believed that by training adequately the hind legs the forehand could be relieved somewhat from its workload. However, studies have shown that this seems not to be feasible and it even appears that in stronger collection there is greater force on the forehand. In fact the back and abdominal muscles of the horse need to be trained more. This can be achieved by an increased rounding of the back and a stronger stepping under the body.

Looking at the horse thoroughly, it quickly becomes clear that it has a very strong hind part, which is well suited to round the back upward and bear the weight of the rider. But only if the horse angles the hind legs more and rounds the back upward by putting the legs more under the body.

If the centre of gravity is changed in that way, the horse finds a position to carry the rider without any major health damage. That's why we train dressage with the horse: to enable the horse to carry the rider! This should be considered for every horse, regardless of discipline.

The whole training of the horse is designed to bring the hind legs more to the centre of gravity and thus achieve a greater rounding of the back and getting off more weight bearing from the forehands.

The dressage horse is different to other horses regarding the degree of the collection and the capability of raising the forehand, particularly in the higher movements (such as piaffe, passage). A dressage horse is especially trained for strength. It has relatively thick muscles that can keep the strength for a strong collection in the long run of a competition.

Imagine to lift a barbell: this effort can be only held for a certain time. The more you repeat this exercise, however, the longer you hold the bar, we speak of strength endurance.

Therefore, a dressage horse is visually different from an endurance or eventing horse. The large muscles of a dressage horse would be detrimental in endurance sports because they need much more power and a corresponding cooling.

Nevertheless, the basic work of the horses of different disciplines is the same. They go through the steps of training – gait; suppleness; contact between hand and mouth; impulsion; straightening until the collection. The horses learn to round the back and can then develop from the collecting work a certain muscular power that will put them into a position to bear more weight with the hind legs in order to carry the rider for a long time. To achieve this goal the dressage / gymnastic work is performed with the horse. Previously the dressage training served as training and gymnastic work of the horse in preparation for its job as a riding horse (especially in the military field for endurance), but today only dressage movements are ridden.

The general opinion is that a dressage horse goes M-dressage, when it is able to do flying changes and S-dressage, when it performs piaffe and passage. However, those movements do not say anything about the real level of schooling, but they are used as gymnastic training. A piaffe trains the hind legs of the horse as it represents the highest degree of collection. sidework as travers, tenvers, shoulder-in and half passes encourage the longitudinal flexion of a horse, its softness and the increased load of the respective inner hind leg. But all those movements serve only the training.

Many riders misunderstand the proper riding of a horse by trying among other things to get the horse's head down with the use of sharp bits. They put their horse together by holding the reins and driving massively from behind. The horse avoids the pressure by putting the head down and behind the vertical. Because of this the horse then first blocks and afterwards hollows the back. These riders think their horse would go on the bit, since the optical conditions are indeed met.

The concept of leaning on the bit has nothing to do with keeping the horse's head in a certain position, but it is called as a light, flexible connection between the rider's hand and horse's mouth. The contact between hand and mouth as well as the raising of the forehand must always be seen relative to the degree of collection. The more the hind legs step under the centre of gravity the more the horse raises the head and neck. A loose trotting horse runs in a low raising of the forehand and minimum contact between hand and mouth. A dressage horse doing Passage or Piaffe raises the forehand a lot more depending on the flexion of the hind legs. The contact to the mouth also gets stronger. Both horses have in common, however, that the neck is always the highest point. Only in this position the horse is able to round the back.

The rounding of the back, bringing the hind legs under the body and the increased weight bearing of the hind legs are, independent of the riding, the criteria one should always pay attention for. Only the properly trained and ridden horses will stay sound.

Looking at the technical training it becomes clear, that the back, the sacro-iliac area and the suspensory ligaments (mainly behind) are the most heavily used areas of a dressage horse. The amount of rotation movements the horses have to perform, because of few straight lines and a lot of bending lines, explains the common injuries in a dressage horse. As a veterinarian we should always be aware of the effects of this technical / power training.

Beside the technical and strength training the rider should keep an eye on the endurance training of the dressage horse. We know that a dressage horse performs at an average heart rate of 140-160 beats /min. To improve the endurance capability of the dressage horse, it is enough to do twice a week canter work at a speed of 300-360 m/min for about ten minutes.

The whole dressage training should be a mix of strength (repeating several movements) training and endurance training (canter work twice a week). The secret of a good dressage training is to understand the effects of the technical / strength / power training (hind legs under the centre of gravity, round back, neck highest point in the collection) and to combine it with a sufficient amount of endurance training. The rider should never ask for much rotation movements to a tired horse. That is the moment where the horses get injured because the muscles cannot compensate the forces anymore.

Final discussion

The different ways of Courouce-Malblanc, Lindholm and Croon and Lindner to do performance diagnostics and guide the conditioning of horses based on the results of testing show that there are many ways to provide the service of guiding training by physiological or biochemical parameters, but all methods have the advantage of providing for objective individualization!

The key for improving an athlete as much as possible is to know whether he is reacting adequately to the training program being applied. This is accomplished by the standardized exercise testing (SET). However, different SET prescriptions mean different values of the same parameters measured regardless of these being derived from the blood (plasma) lactate running speed, heart rate running speed or even oxygen consumption speed relationships (so far mainly a treadmill based tool; Rose *et al.*, 1990). These differences are not important as long as the objective of their determination is to diagnose performance. Just stick to one SET prescription, if the repeatability of the values is good. The same holds for guiding the training. However, when the one or another hint of the different authors involved in this article is to be applied, then it is important to realize that the same parameter means a very different value because changing the duration of the steps has a large impact on the lactate concentration in blood (Figure 5). The effect of changing the duration of steps in SETs has a rather small effect on the parameters derived from the HRRS relationship compared to the effects on the blood lactate running speed relation. The reason for this is that heart rate does not reflect duration but speed of exercise only whilst the blood lactate concentration is affected by both exercise parameters. This holds for the range of time of the steps (intervals) of the SETs described in this article.

The effect of changing the duration of the steps in the SET was quantified some years ago (Köster 1996). Horses were submitted in a randomized order on a treadmill set at 6% slope to SETs with steps of 1, 3 and 5 minutes duration (one duration of steps during one SET only). The initial speed was 6 m/s for all SET and speed was increased by 0.5 m/s until horses had a blood lactate concentration of 4 mmol/l or more. In Figure 5 is shown the example of the blood lactate running speed curves of one horse running the SET with steps of differing duration. In the SET with the steps of 1 min duration the horse run 11 steps before reaching 4 mmol/l, in the SET with 3 min steps it run 6, and in the SET with 5 min steps 4 steps. The respective mean v_4 values were 10.5 m/s, 8.2 m/s and 7.5 m/s (Figure 5).

The duration of the steps and intervals of the SETs prescribed by Courouce-Malblanc (3 min) and Croon and Lindholm (variable, always under 5 min and towards the higher speeds even below 2 min at the end) are less than the 5 min steps used by Lindner and colleagues in all the studies presented in Table 1. Thus, it has to be realized that the values of the same BLRS derived parameters obtained with the SETs prescribed by Courouce-Malblanc and Croon and Lindholm are higher than those determined with the SET prescribed by Lindner!

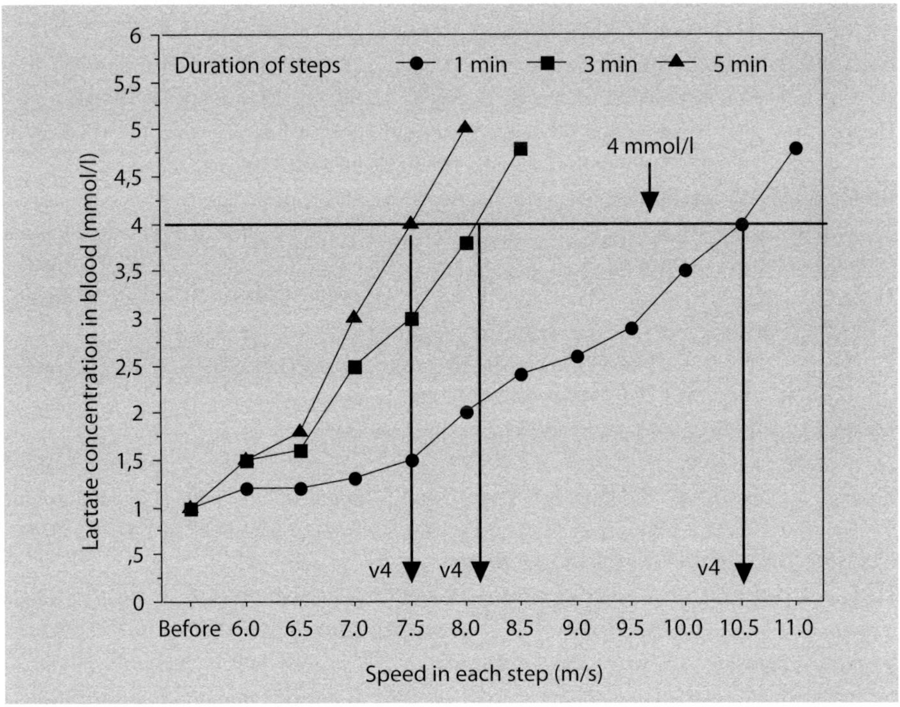

Figure 5. Blood lactate running speed curves of a horse submitted on different days to SETs with steps of 1, 3 and 5 min duration (Köster, 1996).

Hopefully this collaborative effort and the continuous testing done by others to control the effects of the guided training will allow horses to be better prepared to cope with the demands of sports!

References

Amory, H., Art, T., Linden, A., Desmecht, D., Buchet, M., Lekeux, P. (1993) Physiological response to the cross-country phase in eventing horses. J Eq Vet Sci 13: 646-650.

Auvinet, B., Galloux, P., Michaux, J.M., Lepage, O., Franqueville, M.. De Faucompret, J., Ansaloni-Galloux, A., Coureau, C., Goupil, X. (1989) Test d'effort standardisé de terrain pour chevaux de concours complet d'équitation. Médecine et sports équestres, VIIème congrès des pays francophones, Saumur: p. 432-463.

Couroucé, A. (1998) Endurance and sprint training. In Proceedings: Conference on Equine Sports Medicine and Science (CESMAS). p 190-202.

Couroucé, A. (1999) Field Exercise testing for assessing fitness in French Standardbred trotters. Vet J 157: 112-122.

Dag, S. (1998) Trainingsabhängige morphologische Befunde an der Skelettmuskulatur beim Pferd. Doctoral thesis Vet School of Hanover, Germany.

Galloux, P. (1991) Contribution à l'élaboration d'une planification de la préparation énergétique du cheval de concours complet: suivi de l'entraînement par la mesure de la fréquence cardiaque et le dosage de la lactatémie. Thèse de doctorat de l'université de Poitiers, France.

Gansen, S., Lindner, A., Marx, S., Mosen, H., Sallmann, H.P. (1999) Effect of conditioning horses with lactate-guided exercise on muscle glycogen content. Eq. Vet. J. Suppl 30: 329-331.

Hasson, O. (1994) Comparaison de deux epreuves d´effort standardise chez des chevaux de concourse complet. These de doctoratde la faculte de medecine de Creteil, France.

Köster, A. (1996) Reproducibility of performance parameters of horses derived from standardized exercise tests (v_2, v_3, v_4, v_{12}, v_{150}, v_{180}, v_{200}) on treadmill and the effect of duration of step and length of interval. Doctoral thesis for veterinary medicine, University of Giessen, Germany.

Leleu, C., Cotrel, C., Couroucé-Malblanc, A. (2005) Relationships between physiological variables and race performance in French standardbred trotters. Vet Rec 156: 339-342.

Lindner, A. (2000) Use of blood biochemistry for positive performance diagnosis of sport horses in practice. Rev. Med. Vet. 151:611-618.

Lindner, A. (2010) Relationships between racing times of Standardbreds and v_4 and v_{200}. J. J Anim Sci 2010, 88: 950-954.

Lindner, A., Lopez, R.A., Miranda, R.P., Desmarás, E., Boffi, F.M. (2007) Effect of conditioning horses 2 x week with exercise at v_{10} on v_4. In: Scientific proceedings of Voorjaarsdagen, Amstedam, The Netherlands. p. 260.

Lindner, A., López, R.A., Durante, E., Ferreira, V., Boffi, F.M. (2009a) Effect of conditioning horses 3 times a week with exercises at v_{10}. J Eq Vet Sci 2009, 29: 828-832.

Lindner, A., Mosen, H., Kissenbeck, S., Fuhrmann, H., Sallmann, H.P. (2009b) Effect of blood lactate-guided conditioning of horses with exercises of differing duration and intensities on heart rate and biochemical blood variables. J. Anim. Sci. 87, 3211-3217.

Persson, S.G.B. (1983) Evaluation of Exercise Tolerance and Fitness in the Performance Horse. In: Equine Exercise Physiology I, Eds: D.H. Snow, S.G.B. Persson, R.J. Rose. Burlington Press, (Cambridge) Ltd., Foxton, Cambridge. p. 470-486.
Rivero, J.L.L., Ruz, A., Marti-Korff, S., Lindner, A. (2006) Contribution of exercise intensity and duration to training-linked myosin transitions in Thoroughbreds. Eq. Vet. J. Suppl 36: 311-315.
Rivero, J.L.L., Ruz, A., Marti-Korff, S., Estepa, J.C., Aguilera-Tejero, E., Werkmann, J., Sobotta, M., Lindner, A. (2007) Effects of intensity and duration of exercise on muscular responses to training of Thoroughbred racehorses. J. Appl. Physiol. 102: 1871-1882.
Trilk, J.L., Lindner, A., Greene, H.M., Alberghina, D., Wickler, S.J. (2002) A lactate-guided conditioning program to improve endurance performance. Eq. Vet. J. Suppl 34: 122-125.
Van Erck, E., De Moffarts, B., Art, T., Lekeux, P. (2005) Evaluation de la condition sportive du cheval de complet sur le terrain. In: Proceedings of AVEF, Angers, 469.
Werkmann, J., Lindner, A., Sasse, H.H. (1996) Conditioning effects in horses of exercise of 5, 15 or 25 minutes´duration at two blood lactate concentrations. Pferdeheilkunde 12: 474-479.

How to evaluate performance of show jumpers before, during and after the competitive season

Philippe Benoit
Clinique Equine, 4 Route de Vilpert, 78610 Les Breviares, France

As a practitioner, and after reading a few articles about performance evaluation, I try to focus on a simple test that I can do in the field with for sure some constraints because conditions change often. Nevertheless, here is my point about show jumpers:

- Show jumpers nowadays do train and show on similar footing, most of the time heavy wet sand, non penetrating and quite firm.
- They practice mostly at canter.
- Their riders at high level have a similar attitude when it is time to look at them on the flat.

My aim was to reduce the number of parameters that may affect the evaluation of the results. Thus, I do a short exercise test with work of 15 minutes duration after warm up (T1). The horses then gallop for 3 minutes at 3 speeds: at 350 m/min (T2), at 450 (T3), and 550 m/min (T4). Between each step the horse walks for 1 min. I take blood and check heart rate in between each step, and check essentially venous lactate, and at the end CPK / AST which can be repeated the next day.

Then I have an idea on how the general condition of the horse is.

I do the exercise test always when horses who have no real clinical findings, do suffer from poor performance or do not recover well from exercise and competition.

In the jumping discipline, poor performance is mostly related to:

- Subclinical lung disease: bleeders that do not jump as good the last fences of a parcours, cough at the exit of the class, or later (may or not may bleed).
- Horses with deep airway disease who have a hard time to recover before a jump off, or a second round.
- Upper airway disease is most of the time well tolerated in my experience because the type of exercise is short (anaerobic) and we can train these horses with a good interval system.
- Abnormal heart auscultation: could have an effect on fitness, but can be better assessed on a treadmill and echocardiography.
- Musculoskeletal pathologies: mostly back problems and related muscle spasms.
- Chronic front feet pain.

Curiously a number of sources of moderate lameness seen do not generate pain when the horse warms up and jumps!

On a show ground, I may repeat the test and measure blood lactate and heart rate just before and after the test or an exercise session.

I expect during this test or exercise session that the horse does not exceed 180 heart beats/min and 4.5 mmol/l of lactate. The heart rate normally comes down to less than 90 during the 1 min phase at walk between steps.

When lactate is higher than that, especially over 7 mmol/l, I will suspect lung subclinical problems or bleeders, minor immune system depression (viral infection), early muscle spasms 'tying up' that I would correlate with the CPK values.

I take seriously even a small increase of CPK (>500) if the horse is normally always under 400 U/l after showing (method of measurement should for sure be the same).

When the heart rate is higher than 180, especially during the 2nd step or after an exercise session, I would suspect first a lack of fitness, and a musculoskeletal source of pain.

A combination of both (lactate and heart rate values increased) is for me definitely a lack of physical fitness.

This test has for sure a lot of weaknesses, but I like to share it with you to eventually improve it.

Prepurchase exam of the high level jumper

Philippe Benoit
Clinique Equine des Bréviaires, 78610 Les Breviaires, France

Aims

The pre purchase exam is a very specific type of examination which aim is to determine if a particular horse is able to participate to a certain type of work or competition. In this topic, my service is to examine the horse supposed to participate in high level competition as a jumper.

- The horse has to be sound to compete at the expected level.
- The horse needs to have a good physical exam and musculoskeletal status if needed to be sold.
- The horse with its potential problem will have to be managed in a certain environment that we need as practitioner to evaluate (stabling, training, footing, shoeing…).

The problem is to assess a horse of which we have no or limited prior knowledge. Our service as vet practitioners will be to evaluate the risk of a purchase and give our client a way of managing the horse after the decision of purchase. This will end up as a more detailed and specific type of exam.

I will go through all the steps of a conventional exam adding specific tests and enquiries that should be evaluated to give a final comment to the potential buyer.

The practitioner will have to make an enquiry to get a maximum amount of information in a small amount of time.

If possible:

- Communicate with other professionals who dealed before with the horse: the veterinarian, the farrier, the physiotherapist, the trainer, the rider.
- Access previous clinical records, medical images, videos.
- Find competition records and check dates to see if there are gaps of time in between suspecting rest or injuries.
- Try to know what the horse has been living with.

Looking at the passport

- Check vaccination record in agreement with national law and FEI rules.
- Check number and frequency of shows the horse participated in.
- For ponies, make sure that the withers height is correct under national or FEI rules.

Static exam

- Medical / Internal part
  1. Heart auscultation has to be rigorous even if most of the heart pathologies (exception of major heart rhythm pathologies as atrial fibrillation) are well tolerated by jumpers.
  2. Special care of the lung auscultation should be done since a few diseases including EIPH (use of endoscopy and Xrays) are definitely affecting performance. Upper respiratory problems such as roaring are affecting partially only the condition but would be a challenge in case of resale.
- Teeth evaluation because they are part of most of the behaviour induced problems, and may interfere with other sources of neck and back pain as well as misbehaviour.
- Orthopaedic / conformation: there have been a few attempts to find a relation between physical conformation and ability of jumping with poor success. Nevertheless, there are a few findings we prefer not to have for the high level competition:
  1. Extreme defect of front feet weight bearing (toe in or toe out) and long pastern low fetlock axis on front or hinds as they are known to promote a real risk of suspensory ligament strain and lesion.
  2. Muscling should be as symmetric as possible. Special observation will be given to base of withers, low neck and especially gluteus area.
  3. Some joints may be mildly effusive with no significant clinical relation unless passive flexion tests are positive (painful as the horse is standing).

Dynamic exam

As usual, the dynamic exam starts on a straight line and on a figure 8 at the walk where maximum attention is given to the way the horse bends sideways and the axial skeleton should align itself naturally to the curve. This will give ideas of any areas of defect of motion between the top of the neck to the tail. Each fetlock should drop (overextend) equally.

At the trot on straight line and circles, the horse is examined with special interest to the back motion which should be evaluated sideways and from behind. For sure any source of discomfort, including defect of cranial phase or caudal phase of the stride will be noticed.

High level jumper may show extraordinary length of stride, and some hyperextension of the front / hind limbs movement that should be differentiated from moderate uncoordination. On the circle, again, same attention is given to bending at trot and canter. Every part of the body should move fluently as a 'wave'. The canter should be giving a good 3 beat with nice suspension phase. The horse should remain perpendicular to the ground on a lunge line and not leaning inside (more characteristic of lumbosacral type of pain). The horse can be sound but have trouble to maintain a nice equivalent and symmetric stride from one side to the other. Therefore, a horse who does not hold the lead, counter canters, or has a moderate dissociation of both hinds might be suspected of having hind limb subclinical problems that may not show up in a conventional exam.

The surcingle test (Desbrosse) gives a good idea of potential thoracic pain or longissimus spasms.

Dynamic flexion tests are mandatory and should be negative for most of this high level sport horses. A comparison of the weight and ease to flex should be compared with the findings of the static exam to evaluate potential improvement due to the warm up.

Dynamic hoof test is systematically done in our practice to underline any source of local heel pain as the horse jogs (even more significant when a horse shows a shorter stride circling on hard footing).

Exam under tack

Such high level horses should be seen under tack. There are nevertheless 2 problems due to the fact of asking the horse to be ridden by another person than the official rider, or having a professional insurance that does not cover this type of demand which is not widely accepted. But, this exam, is in my opinion, a very interesting exam to pick up subtle lameness or asymmetry when changing reins. This exercise may help to understand subtle abnormality that the horse may exacerbate once he competes at the highest level.

The protocol is always the same having the horse in a light frame on a large figure 8 at the trot, and the rider is asked to change lead of diagonal to see the change in the weight bearing of each 4 limbs. We found per example this test very relevant to pick up early stifle or suspensory sources of discomfort as the rider is loading with the inside limb (fore or hind).

With the same idea, it is very interesting to watch videos of the horse performing and note any source of abnormality such as:

- landing on a preferred limb;
- defect of bending of one part of the back between fences or over the fence;
- defect of canter stride (length, disunited, gait) from left to right;
- difficulty to collect in between fences.

After dynamic exam, I am willing to palpate and manipulate the back, neck, flexor tendons and major joints to look for any source of pain, distension and differences with my earlier findings when the horse was cold and standing.

All the information collected after this full clinical examination should lead to list the good and bad points of the horse itself and try to make a hierarchy of problems according to the type of discipline.

At this stage, even if imaging including at least Xrays and ultrasound exams are done, there is a need to make sure, especially for older horses to understand that abnormal findings on the clinical exam and imaging techniques should be matching so the practitioner can give at least a potential diagnosis but also a prognosis when possible.

This again will put the practitioner in a more critical position where he may advice a follow up procedure to maintain the horse in the sport.

Xray exam

Most of the normal Xray check ups have been already described in many lectures. There are a few possibilities to create a standard amount of pictures. Our aim again is to obtain a maximum amount of information with a minimum of Xrays. In most of these check up I may prefer to have views of the neck, back, and splint bones to confirm or document my clinical exam instead of always repeating the conventional battery of xray images.

From the standard protocol involving all the distal joints, I may certainly ask for low neck and mid back Xrays, which could be completed with ultrasound imaging.

Ultrasonography

This type of imaging should be done each time the horse is more than 7 years old and already competes at high level. Younger horses, also depending on the amount of transaction, should get scanned some ligament and tendon structures. I normally examine the following structures:
- Suspensory ligament (proximal area) of all limbs almost systematically.
- Suspensory distal branches, SDFT and fetlock ligaments especially on long pastern low fetlock conformation horses.
- Neck cervical epiaxial joints evaluation on stiff neck horses, or showing light uncoordination.

- Back: Thoraco-lumbar area and epiaxial lumbar joints externally, and if pelvis motion is poor and if both parties agree, I would propose internal rectal evaluation of sacro-iliac and lumbosacral joints.

Endoscopy

When vetting high level performers in show jumping, it is quiet easy to have access to videos or trials of the client or usual rider. Therefore, if the horse is a roarer or has an abnormal noise during exercise, it will be easy to have a quick information and make an upper respiratory tract endoscopy to document this noise. Therefore, if the horse has not shown such pathology and has a normal slap test, I may not, after asking my client and making my own assessment, follow up with an endoscopy. This also means on the contrary, that any abnormal finding, including respiratory auscultation, should be leading the practitioner to make an endoscopy.

Gastroscopy

This type of exam is even more invasive than the previous type of endoscopy. Therefore, it is not done on a systematic base. We should try to have enough information from previous owner/s and all professionals surrounding the horse to know if the horse has been suffering from gastritis and/or ulcers. This disease appears to be significantly responsible of many poor performance issues and we see in our experience horses suffering from chronic back pain with related gastritis. Subsequently, I may try to obtain the authorization from the owner to do this exam in the near future (before transaction) if there is any high suspicion during the prepurchase clinical exam.

This is one of this exams that you may ask to be done as complementary to document a clinical suspicion and give your client maximum information before the final transaction.

Other type of imaging

MRI and Bone Scan are being already done in a few scenarios of prepurchase exams. There is nevertheless a barrier to be established to avoid such exams, unless the practitioner needs a very precise information in order to help his client making a very fine decision.

When it comes to such exam, it is more to fail the horse, which most of the vets can definitively do by doing a very thorough clinical exam and therefore avoid undertaking this type of medical imaging.

I would consider essentially the case of a horse which has been injured, and comes for sale with a good documentation, eventually with MRI images, that may need such an imaging to track or prove a specific healing process or the stabilisation of a known lesion (bone oedema, cartilage thinning, ligament strain…) before the decision for transaction.

Blood work

High level jumpers are subject to travel far from home, and may also be resold in foreign countries where certain serology must be negative. For all horses, I will ask for a Coggins test. For stallion and high potential mares, I may propose my clients to do a CEM swap. For any other horses, especially travelling, or sold to USA and competing overseas, you must do a piroplasmosis serology test.

Finally, I run systematically a blood cell count and a standard biochemistry. Medication tests are also done on whole blood, even if we are aware that we will pick up only recently used drugs, and these tests will include anti-inflammatory drugs, sedatives, bronchodilatators and steroids.

Conclusion

The prepurchase exam of the high level jumper is like a police enquiry which starts with the collection of a great amount of information around the history, and performance record of the horse. The practitioner, besides doing a normal standard exam, shall go in some more specific clinical tests and imaging procedures to document some of the most challenging patterns that are difficult to manage.

Our role is to identify the good and poor sides of the horse in order to maintain the horse in the sport, or to be sold again if we are dealing with professional riders or dealers. Therefore, it becomes a challenge to list the problems of the horse giving our own hierarchy to be able to offer a very individual and specific management. This shall be done in agreement with our knowledge of the future rider and professional environment, which includes the stabling, the training, and all the individuals working as a team with the vet practitioner.

References

Andrews, J. (2005) Gastric ulcers in horses J Anim Sci 83, 18-21.

Benoit, P. (2006) How to make a specific examination of the jumper, in Proceedings Assoc. American Equine Practitioner, San Antonio, USA.

Boswell, R., Mitchell, R., Dyson, S. (2003) Lameness in the show hunter and show jumper. In: Ross M.W. and Dyson S.J., eds. Diagnosis and Management of Lameness in the Horse, St. Louis: Saunders, pp 965-975

Château, H., Degeurce, C., Denoix, J.M. (2005) Influence de la nature du sol et de la ferrure sur la biomécanique des articulations digitales, Proc de la 31ème journée de la Recherche Equine, 35-44.

Denoix, J.M. (1999) Spinal biomechanics and functional anatomy. Vet Clin North Am 15, 27-60.

Denoix, J.M. (2008) Biomecanique du cheval de CSO, in Proc Assoc Vét Eq Française, Reims, France.

Denoix, J.M., Dyson, S.J. (2003) The thoracolumbar spine. In: Ross MR and Dyson SJ, eds. Diagnosis and lameness in Horses. Saint Louis, WB Saunders, 509-521.

Dyson, S., Benoit, P. (2008) in Proceedings, CESMAS, Utrecht.

Jeffcott, L.B. (1980) Disorders of the thoracolumbar spine of the horse – a survey of 443 cases. Eq Vet J 12, 197-210.

Mitchell, R.D. (2001) Prevalence of gastric ulcers in hunter/jumper and dressage horses evaluated for poor performance. Association for Equine Sports Medicine.

Body condition scoring and on-track performance diagnosis

B.D. Nielsen
Dept. Animal Science, Michigan State University, East Lansing, MI 48824-1225, USA

There are many factors that play a role in why a horse fails to perform up to expectations. The first, and probably the most common, is that the expectations for the horse were unreasonable. Despite having outstanding bloodlines, a horse may not have the genetics to perform well. This is not surprising as the heritability of many traits associated with performance is typically less than 0.5 for racehorses (Thiruvenkadan *et al.*, 2009a,b). Thus, just because the parents were exceptional performers is no guarantee their offspring are genetically capable of performing at the same level. However, if a horse has been performing well and then that performance begins to decline, various factors can play a role and one of those factors is the nutrition of the animal.

Often when a horse fails to perform up to expectations, the response is to blame the feed the horse is receiving. Many times what is being fed is both adequate and appropriate but there are many times when such is not the case. While many individuals tend to look for problems with the minor portions of the diet such as vitamins or minerals, in truth, their focus should be on a much more critical aspect of the feeding program.

The biggest nutritional difference between exercising and non-exercising horses is the increased energy demands that are typically associated with exercise. While a short-term inadequacy of the intake of most nutrients will not have a noticeable impact on a horse's performance, a horse that does not regularly consume an adequate amount of energy will fatigue faster and not perform as well compared to one that is consuming sufficient quantities. What frequently determines how a horse performs in competition is how quickly it fatigues (Worth, 1985). While there are many biochemical and physiological reasons why fatigue occurs, one of the reasons is a depletion of glycogen stores that could be used to generate energy. Some research has suggested ways to increase glycogen stores through dietary manipulation such as feeding diets containing elevated amounts of oil or fat (Potter *et al.*, 1992; Geelen *et al.*, 2001), but before a person starts to worry about which form of dietary energy is needed, it is important that they simply determine if their horse is receiving enough dietary energy.

Determining whether requirements are being met for most nutrients is difficult without analyzing the diet and comparing the contents of the diets to the animal's nutritional requirements. However, it is possible to evaluate whether energy requirements are being met simply by examining the animal. Some individuals suggest that an animal's behavior can indicate if they are getting too much energy in their diets or the wrong type of energy (for example, some people consider corn to be a 'hot' feed and causes their animals to be unruly). Behavior problems involving an unruly horse are more often related to a horse not enjoying the work it is being asked to do – often because of a training or soreness issue. In contrast, a horse that has a 'lack of energy' and seems sluggish certainly might not be receiving enough calories to meet its energy demands.

Rather than relying on behavior and attitude to determine if energy requirements are being met without being exceeded, a better method is simply to body condition score (BCS) the horse. The BCS can be a useful way to determine if the horse is meeting its caloric requirements without exceeding them. A horse that has a decreasing BCS is using more calories than it is taking in and a horse that has an increasing BCS is taking in more calories than it is using. This is the simplest and probably best way to see if you are meeting the energy requirements.

Even if a horse's BCS is not increasing or decreasing, it does not mean that the animal is at the ideal BCS. For instance, a horse can be at a constant BCS but that BCS could be too high or too low. A commonly used body condition scoring system presented by Henneke *et al.* (1983) is based on a nine-point scale where a 1 represents an emaciated horse and a 9 is an obese individual. An even more detailed version of that system is provided by Schramme (2003). A BCS between 4 and 6 should be the goal for most athletic horses (Becvarova *et al.*, 2009) as some research has suggested that glycogen stores are not maximized when horses are in a thin condition (Jones *et al.*, 1992; Scott *et al.*, 1992). Simply put, the 'gas tank is not full'. Considering glycogen is a preferred substrate for energy production during short-term, high-intensity anaerobic exercise such as in Thoroughbred racing, cutting, or jumping, having a 'full gas tank' will allow the horse to perform for a longer time without slowing down. As the duration or length of competition increases, there is reason to believe that a somewhat lower BCS could be an advantage. During most equine competitions, there is insufficient time to mobilize significant amounts of body fat stores for energy. As a result, higher body fat stores act simply as additional weight that the animal needs to carry around without providing much benefit in terms of immediate energy supply. That is why it is not uncommon to see endurance horses competing at distances of 100 miles or greater with a BCS under a 5 and still doing quite well as compared to ones that have a greater BCS (Lawrence *et al.*, 1992). Similarly, the body mass index (the system that suggests what an ideal weight is for a given height) of elite human marathon runners would be considered to be low by most standards – though obviously having such a low body fat content does not impair the performance of those distance runners.

Slight over-consumption of most nutrients (but not so much as to cause a toxicity) can simply be wasteful and usually is unlikely to impair performance. However, regularly consuming too much dietary energy will likely result in excessive fat deposition. That extra body fat can certainly be detrimental to performance. A horse that is greater than a BCS of 5 is carrying around extra weight and that will impair the performance of most athletic horses. For example, a Thoroughbred racehorse at 500 kg with a BCS of 6 probably weighs about 16 to 20 kg more than a similar-built horse at a BCS of 5. Thus, it is easy to imagine what a difference that could make to its race performance. Other issues that arise because of horses being too fat include an increased risk of injury due to the extra weight they carry causing greater forces on their legs. Additionally, the extra fat serves as insulation and makes it challenging for the horse to dissipate heat (Morgan, 1997). While running out of substrate to generate energy is one reason horses fatigue, overheating is another. When muscle temperatures get too high, enzymes involved in muscle contraction no longer work as efficiently – effectively limiting how much work the animal can do. While carrying extra fat is beneficial to animals living in the arctic because of its insulating properties, it certainly can decrease the performance of an athletic horse. As previously mentioned, muscle glycogen seems to decrease when a horse is thin, but it does not seem to increase when a horse progresses from a moderate BCS to a fat BCS. Thus, there is seemingly little benefit to athletic horses to be much above a BCS of 5. In contrast, one could make an argument that some horses do fine having a BCS a bit lower than a 5 – especially if the distance they compete at is great enough. That being said, it is often a challenge to get enough calories into those hard working horses and it is not being suggested that one try to restrict the feed given to athletic horses in order to achieve a BCS much less than 5 as that certainly could impair performance.

When it comes to nutritional requirements, meeting the energy requirements of athletic horses can be much more challenging than meeting the requirements for other nutrients. It is quite simple to meet the requirements for protein, minerals, or vitamins simply by altering what you feed the horse or supplementing more of those nutrients into their ration. However, with energy, often a horse cannot consume enough calories to meet their energy needs, particularly with a high forage diet (Harris, 2009). Unfortunately, not providing enough dietary energy can have a relatively immediate impact on performance. The positive thing is that energy is the one nutritional requirement where one only needs to monitor their animal to see if the dietary energy intake is matching the energy expenditure. If they match, and if the BCS is in the appropriate range, it increases the chance that your horse will perform well.

Though one should always be cautious about believing anecdotal evidence, a classic example of the influence of inadequate dietary energy intake can have on performance occurred during a visit to Ohi Race Course in Tokyo, Japan. The day before doing a stable visit, I was asked to evaluate the diet a trainer was feeding his small group of horses. It was September and the trainer had not had a winner since opening his stable in April. Comparing the estimated calories provided by the feed to the requirements of the horses, it seemed obvious that the horses were simply not being fed enough calories. Upon visiting the stable and seeing the horses, the BCS of his animals confirmed what we had calculated – his horses were not receiving enough energy. The recommendation was made to feed more (which was seemingly viewed with skepticism as I was accompanying a feed dealer). Fortunately, he acted on the advice and by the end of November all of his horses had won.

The point of this is to not suggest that having the right BCS will make every horse a winner, but to remind that having too low or too high of a BCS can make every horse a loser.

References

Becvarova, I., Pleasant, R.S., Thatcher, C.D. (2009) Clinical assessment of nutritional status and feeding program in horses. Vet Clin N Amer 25, 1-21.

Geelen, S.N., Sloet van Oldruitenborgh-Oosterbaan, M.M., Beyen, A.C. (2001) Supplemental fat in the diet of horses…is it advantageous? Tijdschr Diergeneeskd. 126, 310-315.

Harris, P.A. (2009) Feeding management of elite endurance horses. Vet Clin Equine 25, 137-153

Henneke, D.R., Potter, G.D., Kreider, J.L., Yeates, B.F. (1983) Relationship between condition score, physical measurements and body fat percentages in mares. Eq Vet J 15, 371-372.

Jones, D.L., Potter, G.D., Greene, L.W., Odom, T.W. (19929 Muscle glycogen in exercised miniature horses at various body conditions and fed a control or fat-supplemented diet. J Eq Vet Sci 12, 287-291.

Lawrence, L., Jackson, S., Kline, K., Moser, L., Powell, D., Biel, M. (1992) Observations on body weight and condition of horses in a 150-mile endurance ride. J Eq Vet Sci 12, 320-324.

Morgan, K. (1997) Thermal insulance of peripheral tissue and coat in sport horses. J Therm Biol 22, 169-175

Potter, G.D., Hughes, S.L., Julen, T.R., Swinney, S.L. (1992) A review of research on digestion and utilization of fat by the equine. Pferdeheilkunde. Sonderheft 1, 119-123.

Schramme, C.S. (2003) Body Condition Scores und biometrische Daten zur Abschätzung des Körpergewichtes bei Warmblutpferden. Doctoral thesis Vet Med Ludwig-Maximilians-Universität München

Scott, B.D., Potter, G.D., Greene, L.W., Hargis, P.S., Anderson, J.G. (1992) Efficacy of a fat-supplemented diet on muscle glycogen concentrations in exercising Thoroughbred horses maintained in varying body conditions. J Eq Vet Sci 12, 109-113.

Thiruvenkadanm, A.K., Kandasamy, N., Panneerselvam, S. (2009a) Inheritance of racing performance of Thoroughbred horses. Livestock Sci 121, 308-326.

Thiruvenkadanm, A.K., Kandasamy, N., Panneerselvam, S. (2009b) Inheritance of racing performance of trotter horses: An overview. Livestock Sci 124, 163-181.

Worth, M. (1985) Muscle fatigue in the horse: a review. J Eq Vet Sci 5, 276-278.

The prepurchase examination of horses in Germany

B. Nolting
Tierärztliche Praxis für Pferde, Dr. Björn Nolting GmbH, Heimerzheimer Str. 18, 53919 Weilerswist, Germany

Until 2002 the purchase of horses in Germany was settled by Germanic law. It was purchased as-is. Basically it was a handshake business. Defects were governed by the Imperial Regulation of 1899. On the shortcomings were cribbing, weaving, roaring, glanders, staggers and chronic uveitis.

If a buyer of the horse detected one of these deficiencies within 14 days of a purchase, the purchase was cancelled. In addition only the fraud and the guaranteed properties were regulated in the Penal Code. In these cases the purchase was also cancelled.

In 2002 Germany implemented the new consumer protection law in accordance with the requirements of the European Union. Thus the purchase of horses was now regulated under Roman law. From now on the purchased horses must meet a certain property if it is used for a particular purpose.

At first the new introduced law in Germany led to a large uncertainty. Suddenly the buyers were granted more rights and it was much easier to claim now. At once salesmen were faced with the situation that they were liable for the constitution of the horse at least one year or -without any special appointment- for two years.

In the first years the new legal situation led to many disputes. The lawyers reassured only in few cases and pointed to the expected judgements of the courts and how they would deal with the modified statutory basis. In fact the living horse has been equalised to an object, e.g. a car where defects 'could be fixed by changing spare parts'. Thus, the legal environment changed for the German veterinarians at once.

The big problem with the purchase examination of a horse is, that the German veterinarian does not work in a service contract, where he only provides a proper medical service in accordance with the medical art, without success, but he owes as a consultant a contract for services with success.

For the German veterinarians, there was only one way out of the dilemma. It had to develop a standard procedure. This was done by the horse society. The purchase examination of the horse is divided into a clinical part, a X-ray part and further investigations. The procedures are standardised and documented in a protocol. In particular, to the X-ray examination is given much time. A quality standard, the standard projections and a catalogue of X-ray findings were developed.

The standard projections are:
- side view of the lower limb (coffin, pastern, fetlock) of all 4 legs;
- both front navicular bones (Oxspring technique);
- ap view of the Tarsus and both oblique projections.

Recently were added:
- side view of the stifle;
- back.

However, there is no top on the number of X-rays that can be taken.

In order to assist all veterinarians in the evaluation of the radiographs, the most common radiographic findings have been catalogued in the so-called X-ray guidance. In it, the most common radiographic findings are listed, evaluated and classified according to their health impact. This X-ray guide should allow for the veterinarian to give a 'neutral' opinion on the findings of the X-ray images. By this a common language and assessment are possible. Even lawyers should be able to assess the findings legally through this classification.

X-ray guide 2007

For evaluating the findings in the X-ray images, a classification in four classes is available.
- Class I
  Radiographically without specific findings, and findings that are classified as anatomical shape variations (ideal state).
- Class II
  Results that differ little from the ideal, and for which clinical symptoms can be expected in not more than 3% of the cases within life (Standard status).
- Class III
  Findings, which differ significantly from the norm, and for which clinical symptoms can be expected in about 20% of the cases within life (acceptance condition).
- Class IV
  Findings, which differ significantly from the norm, and for which clinical symptoms are likely (over 50%; risk status).
- Intermediate classes
  Intermediate classes I-II, II-III and III-IV are permitted to address the fact that veterinarians may conclude differently on the same findings according to their experience.

Unfortunately the horse trading and the lawyers declared only horses in classes I and II in principle for fully sellable. The X-ray guide still enables room for interpretation and there are always reasons for legal disputes. To date this problem is not entirely under control. I personally consider that a reasonable explanation and description of the X-ray findings is much more useful than a mere classification.

A buyer can handle it much better when he learns to deal with findings instead of pure numbers between I and IV. No one knows whether a successful sport horse will be equally successful 6 months after purchase exam. That depends on too many factors.

In my opinion during a purchase exam you should point out to all involved that the results represent only a snapshot. It provides the status quo of a horse, as far as possible.

As a veterinarian, you should force yourself to a standard procedure to overlook any possible findings. The findings must be recorded thoroughly and be subject to an objective assessment.

With all involved a thorough informed consent discussion should be conducted, in which all the results are explained and evaluated. To the best knowledge a certain recommendation can be spoken. However, one should avoid to influence a purchasing decision. This should be made by the buyer taking into account all information themselves. Only he himself can determine whether the money fits the value.

Of course the veterinarian is aware of different loads of the horses depending of different disciplines:

- An old tendon injury should be evaluated more critically in an eventing horse than in a jumping horse.
- The load of the forehand of a jumping horse is higher than of a dressage horse.
- The back, the sacro-iliac area and the suspensory ligaments are more stressed in a dressage horse than in a vaulting horse, etc.

In all my professional years, I have found that an open, honest and objective discussion with all of the people involved in buying a horse, is the best solution and ensures the fewest problems. I use a so-called individual contract (see Appendix 1). With its help, the exact extent of the investigation can be determined.

Appendix 1. Individual contract

BURG MÜGGENHAUSEN
Tierärztliche Praxis für Pferde
DR. BJÖRN NOLTING GMBH

TIERÄRZTLICHE
PRAXIS FÜR PFERDE
Dr. Björn Nolting GmbH

EQUINE PRE-PURCHASE EXAM

CUSTOMER:

HORSE:

BREED: GENDER:

COLOR: DOB: REGISTRATION NO:

EXHIBITS:

- ✓ Exam Guidelines
- ☐ Printed Radiographs
- ☐ RÖNTGENBILDER CD / RADIOGRAPHS ON CD
- ☐ Print-out from Endoscopy
- ☐ PRINT-OUT FROM ULTRASOUND

Tierärztliche Praxis für Dr. Björn Nolting GmbH — Sitz: Weilerswist — Amtsgericht Bonn HRB 14200, Geschäftsführer Björn Nolting — 1

Identification: Horse: , Color: , Breed: , Gender: , DOB.: , Registration No.:

A. CONTRACT:

§ 1 Name................,Street..............., Country....... - PLZ....., City............ („**Customer**") hereby engages the services of the veterinarians at the Tierärztlichen Praxis Dr. Björn Nolting GmbH (**Service Provider**) to perform a pre-purchase exam of the following horse name........, colour.........., breed ...., gender........, DOB: ...., PassNr.:. The customer determines the scope of the examination which is further defined in § 10 Part 1 & Part 2 and § 12. This document is a representation of the complete scope of the examination. Any examination not mentioned here is expressively not part of this contract. Any changes to this contract must be submitted in writing. Before the start of the examination the customer was presented with an information sheet about the pre-purchase examination. One copy of the information sheet is attached to this document.

§ 2 The purpose of the examination is to determine any deficiency in the health status of the horse at the time of the examination. Certain behavioral patterns like weaving and cribbing,, as well as certain health problems such as environmentally influenced chronic bronchitis, some diseases of the upper airways that will only become apparent with very strenuous exercise and allergies, cannot be diagnosed. The scope of this examination does not include the diagnosis of any other faults of the horse classified in Germany as „Mängel" (vices) and does not include the judging of the conformation for purposes of valuation as a breeding animal or usefulness for any athletic performance.

§ 3 The veterinarian is not required to explain the risks that each step in the process of conducting the pre-purchase examination entails as long as the Examination does not exceed the scope that was previously determined (B. I - IV). The customer agrees to all procedures necessary during the pre-purchase examination. The customer hereby also assures that the owner of the horse has given his/her approval.

§ 4 The veterinarian is required to keep confidential all results obtained during the pre-purchase examination. The veterinarian is allowed to discuss the results obtained with the owner and/or buyer/seller (if not the customer) as long as the customer has not expressively denied this. Only the customer is presented with the written summary of the pre-purchase examination. Any distribution of this document to others is allowed only after authorization of the veterinarian.

§ 5 The evaluation of any diagnosis made during the examination (Section C) reflects the personal opinion of the veterinarian to his/her best knowledge. A horse is an individual living being with a constantly changing health and fitness level. No prognosis for the future regarding health, suitability or fitness can be made. The customer alone is responsible for the decision to buy/sell or to abstain from the purchase.

§ 6 The cost for the standard **clinical** examination (without radiographs, etc) is calculated as follows: the **customer** personally and individually determines the value/price of the horse in question. Is this value below **€ 5.000** the cost will be **€ 196,00** (+ tax). **If the value chosen by the customer is higher, then the cost of the pre-purchase exam will be increased by 0.50 % of the indicated value.**
This fee has been negotiated between the customer and the veterinarian/Pferdepraxis in accordance with §§ 7 and 8 of this contract, which deviates from the legally required limit of liability and statute of limitation. The customer has been informed that the liability limit and the statute of limitation can be increased in proportion to the increased value of the horse, for an additional fee.

The value of the horse cannot be changed after the examination has begun.

The customer (see above) or the representative, having completed the Power of Attorney, hereby personally and bindingly declares the value/cost of the above mentioned horse to be:

A) € ____________________ Read and accepted: Signature: ____________________

§ 7 For any mistakes made within the scope of the pre-purchase examination the veterinarian/Pferdepraxis is liable for up to the amount indicated as value/purchase price of the horse, **up to a maximum of € 150.000.** If the customer wishes a higher liability limit, the customer is responsible to inform the Pferdepraxis before the start of the examination and this must be acceptable to the Pferdepraxis. Additions to the contract after the beginning of the examination are invalid. Third parties mentioned by name in the contract are held to the same limit of liability. Other parties are excluded from any right to sue. The court of law is Landgericht Bonn.

§ 8 Any claims that the customer may have against the Pferdepraxis have a statute of limitations of six months from the day of this examination due to the individual nature of this contract.

Read and accepted Signature:________

§ 9 If § 8 becomes invalid, the statute of limitations for any claims from customers against the Pferdepraxis is a maximum of one year from the day of the examination.

Read and accepted Signature:________

Tierärztliche Praxis für Dr. Björn Nolting GmbH — Sitz: Weilerswist — Amtsgericht Bonn HRB 14200, Geschäftsführer Björn Nolting — 2

Identifikation: Horse: , Color: , Breed: , Gender: , DOB.:, Registration No.:

§ 10 Definition of the contract of the examination: Part 1	PRICE IN EURO WITHOUT VAT	Confirmation/ Signature	CONFIRMATION OF ADDITIONS
Clinical examination according to protocol B.I. – B. IV. * the price is calculated from the basic fee of € 196,00 plus 0,5 % of the value/price of the horse (as defined by the customer) if it is €5.000 or higher. If the pre-purchase examination is cancelled prematurely by the customer, only the basic fee is due.	196,00 + 0,5 % of the price/value of the horse*	☐ yes Signature: ________ X	
Standard Radiograph Profile: 12 views, Explanations see Information sheet - lateral view of all four lower limbs; 45 ° view of the navicular bone of both front legs; Oblique views of both hocks (app. 45 ° & app. 115 °) and dorso-plantar view of both hocks.	12 x € 24,00 ** = 288,00	☐ yes Signature: ________ X	
Skyline view of the navicular bone: This special view of the navicular bone allows insight into the flexor surface of the navicular bone. It is possible that the navicular bone looks normal in the 45° view, but shows defects in the skyline view. Highly recommended! ☐ Right Front ☐ Left Front	33,00 / per view	☐ yes Signature: ________ X	
Lateral view of the stifle: Lateral view of the patella and parts of the tibia and femur. ☐ Right Hind ☐ Left Hind	31,00 / per view	☐ yes Signature: ________ X	
Dorso-plantar view of the stifle: Image of the stifle joint with view of the joint space. ☐ Right Hind ☐ Left Hind	31,00 / per view ***	☐ yes Signature: ________ X	
Oblique view of the fetlock joint and sesamoid bones: more detail of the joint surface, status of the sesamoids, potential "chips" or isolated bony changes. ☐ Right Front ☐ Left Front ☐ Right Hind ☐ Left Hind	31,00 / per view ***	☐ yes Signature: ________ X	
Dorso-palmar and dorso-plantar view of the fetlock joint and sesamoid bones: Image of the joint space and the lateral edges of all bones in view. ☐ Right Front ☐ Left Front ☐ Right Hind ☐ Left Hind	31,00 / per view ***	☐ yes Signature: ________ X	
Lateral view of the dorsal spinous processes of the vertebrae from behind the withers to the lumbar vertebrae: In general, good quality images are possible. In case of heavy muscling or adipose tissue the image quality may deteriorate. This view allows the determination of space in-between spinous processes and chronic changes like "kissing spines".	33,00 / per view	☐ yes Signature: ________ X	
More examples of potential radiographic images: Cervical vertebrae, Shoulder joint, Elbow joint, Carpal joint, Splint bones, and more: ☐ Amount:	31,00 / per view ***	☐ yes Signature: ________ X	
Copies of Radiographs (Price/Sheet) generally 4 views per sheet Radiograph-CD (formatted in high definition DICOM, incl. viewing-software)	10,00 /sheet ☐ 18,00/CD ☐	☐ yes Signature: ________ X	

** special price when choosing standard profile, otherwise € 27,00/view; *** special price in conjunction with pre-purchase examinations for images in addition to the standard profile, otherwise € 27,00 /view.

Tierärztliche Praxis für Dr. Björn Nolting GmbH | Sitz: Weilerswist Geschäftsführer Björn Nolting | Amtsgericht Bonn HRB 14200 | 3

Identifikation: Horse: , Color: , Breed: , Gender: , DOB.: , Registration No.:

§ 10 Definition of the contract of the examination : Part 2 :	PRICE IN EURO WITHOUT VAT	Confirmation/ Signature	CONFIRMATION OF ADDITIONS
Endoscopic examination of the larynx and upper airways: Access via nostrils and view of the pharynx, larynx, trachea, and the primary bronchial tree and the septum separating it.	85,00	☐ yes Signature: ____________ X	
Ultrasound examination: View of individual organs. ☐	(from 45,00)	☐ yes Signature : ____________ X	
„Doping-Test", Blood test in the lab of Professor Schänzer, Sporthochschule Köln: ☐ A.) Taking blood and checking it for NSAIDs & Corticosteroids (incl. taking blood and sending it to the lab) ☐ B.) additional check for sedatives (complete check: free and conjugated chemicals) ☐ C.) Taking blood and storage (freezing of serum) for six months ☐ D.) Shipping of special Drug testing set, additional cost: € 35,00 **Check for anabolic steroids only possible from urine after prior arrangement with Pferdepraxis.**	A.) 150,00 B.) 115,00 C.) 45,00 D.) 35,00	☐ A.) Signature: ☐ B.) ☐ C.) ____________ X ☐ D.)	
Lab check: ☐ A.) Big screening ☐ B.) Fecal check for internal parasites ☐ C.) Other:	A.) 64,00 B.) 54,00 C.)	☐ A.) Signature: ☐ B.) ☐ C.) ____________ X	
☐ Breeding soundness examination of the mare / ☐ Breeding soundness examination of the stallion	Price on Demand	☐ yes Signature : ____________ X	
Rectal examination (palpation of the accessible pelvic and abdominal cavity by the examining veterinarian)	39,00	☐ yes Signature : ____________ X	

§ 11 The Pferdepraxis Dr. Björn Nolting GmbH will take and evaluate radiographs made within the scope of the pre-purchase exam. They belong to the Pferdepraxis Dr. Björn Nolting GmbH and copies can be made for an additional fee. The originals will remain in possession of Pferdepraxis Dr. Björn Nolting GmbH. Radiographs submitted by the customer for inclusion in the pre-purchase exam must have been evaluated in writing by the original veterinarian. The Pferdepraxis Dr. Björn Nolting GmbH explicitly states that the evaluation of the radiographs will not be along the guidelines of the **„Röntgenleitfaden" of 31.08.2002** because they are deemed insufficient.

§ 12 Other Agreements:

____

§ 13 Should part of this contract become invalid, the rest will remain in effect. The invalid statement will be replaced with a valid statement that is as close as possible to the meaning of the original statement.

______________, the ________ X____________________ ______________________________

Place Date Customer Examining veterinarian (Pferdepraxis Dr. Björn Nolting GmbH)

Tierärztliche Praxis für Dr. Björn Nolting GmbH | Sitz: Weilerswist Geschäftsführer Björn Nolting | Amtsgericht Bonn HRB 14200 | 4

Identifikation: Horse: , Color: , Breed: , Gender: , DOB.: , Registration No.:

B. Examination Guidelines:

B. 1. History: Declaration by Seller/Representative

Name: ______________________ Address: ______________________

Phone: ______________________ ______________________

Duration of ownership / possession of horse since: ______________________

Performance of a pre-purchase examination in the last 12 weeks: ☐ yes Results: ____________ ☐ no ☐ unknown ;

Use of horse/ Training status of the horse: ☐ Dressage_______ ☐ Jumping_______ ☐ Cross Country _____

☐ Western_______ ☐ Racing (Galopping) _______ ☐ Leisure ☐ Just started/Green ☐ Other: _______

Use in the last 6 weeks: ☐ Sport ☐ Training ☐ Stall rest ☐ Pasture

Medications in the last 6 weeks: ☐ no ☐ yes: ______________________

Earlier Lameness: ______________________

Earlier Diseases:

____

Surgeries: ☐ Castration; ______________________

____

Behavioral problems (Weaving, Cribbing, etc.): ______________________

Horse kept in: ☐ Stall ☐ Pasture ☐ Open stall with pasture access ☐ Stall & Pasture

Feeding: ☐ Hay ☐ dry ☐ wet ; ☐ Silage ☐ Oats ☐ Pellets ☐ Sweet Feed ☐ other:

Stall bedding material: ☐ Straw ☐ Shavings ☐ Other:

____

Last shoeing: ______________________ Last deworming: ______________________

Vaccination: ☐ regularly ☐ Influenza ☐ Rhino/Herpes ☐ Tetanus Toxoid ☐ Others:

Horse passport: ☐ present FEI-Passport: ☐ present Medication slip (in passport): ☐ present ☐ Slaughter ☐ Non-slaughter

I hereby declare to the best of my knowledge and conscience that all statements made are complete and correct. I agree to all procedures necessary in connection with the pre-purchase exam. This includes the taking of blood for purposes of a drug test, sedation, if necessary, for an endoscopic exam and the removal of the shoes for the radiographic exam of the navicular bone. I will / will not* be present personally for the pre-purchase examination.

Mr./Mrs. ____________________ from ____________________ is hereby authorized to sign all paperwork in my absence.

Signer is: ☐ Owner ☐ Seller ☐ Authorized representative

______________, the ________ X______________________

Place Date Signature (Seller or Owner or Authorized representative)

* Strike non-applicable information

Tierärztliche Praxis für
Dr. Björn Nolting GmbH

Sitz: Weilerswist

Amtsgericht Bonn HRB 14200
Geschäftsführer Björn Nolting

5

Identifikation: **Horse:** , **Color:** , **Breed:** , **Gender:** , **DOB.:** , **Registration No.:**

B.2. ☐ Client ☐ Buyer ☐ Seller

Name: ....

Address: ....

.... -......................

B. 3. ☐ Buyer ☐ Seller ☐ see. B.1

Name: ______________________________

Address: ______________________________

____

Telephone: ______________________________

B. 4. Third Party as per § 7 of the contract:

Name: ______________________________ Address: ______________________________

Phone: ______________________________ ______________________________

B. 5. Persons present during the pre-purchase exam:

☐ Buyer☐ Seller ☐ Third Party/B.4. ; ______________________________

B. 6. Place and Day of pre-purchase exam:

☐ Burg Müggenhausen, the ______________ or ☐______________ , the ___________

B. 7. History: Declaration of Buyer/Representative:

The horse was test-ridden before the pre-purchase exam: ☐ no ☐ yes

Obvious abnormalities: ☐ no ☐ yes ______________________________

B. 8. Signalement of the horse:

Name: Registration Number/Passport:

Breed: Gender:

DOB/Age(Teeth/Papers): ; ______ Color: /______

☐ Instead of Signalment , see copy of equine passport attached.

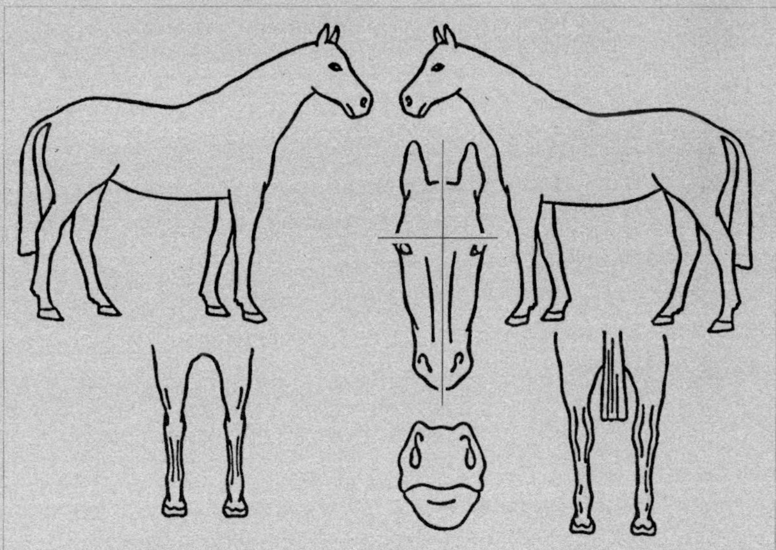

Tierärztliche Praxis für Dr. Björn Nolting GmbH Sitz: Weilerswist Amtsgericht Bonn HRB 14200 Geschäftsführer Björn Nolting 6

Identification: Horse: , Color: , Breed: , Gender: , DOB.: , Registration No.:

B. I. General Examination

Diagram to draw Scars, Splints, obvious abnormalities:
→ Scars O Splints + Other

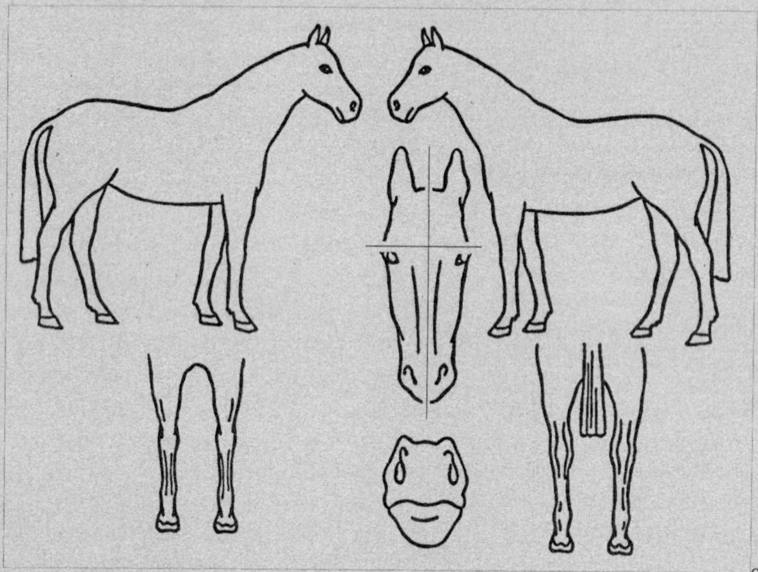

Care/State of Nutrition: ☐ normal ____
Skin and Coat: ☐ normal ____
Obvious Scars: ☐ no ____
General Behavior: ☐ normal ____
Rectal Temperature (when questionable): ____ °C
Pulse: Resting: ____ / min. Quality: ☐ normal ____
Auscultation of the Heart: ☐ normal ____
Respiratory system: Resting frequency: ____ / min.
Breathing: ☐ normal ☐ labored Inhalation ☐ labored Exhalation
Nasal discharge: ☐ no ____
Spontaneous coughing: ☐ no ____
Inducible coughing: ☐ no ____
Palpation of larynx: ☐ normal ____
Auscultation of trachea: ☐ normal ____
Palpation of trachea: ☐ normal ____
Auscultation of lung: ☐ normal ____
After forced deep breaths ☐ normal ____
Mucous membranes: ☐ normal ____
Conjunctiva: ☐ normal ____
Mandibular lymph nodes: ☐ normal ____
Jugular veins: ☐ normal ____

Tierärztliche Praxis für Dr. Björn Nolting GmbH — Sitz: Weilerswist — Amtsgericht Bonn HRB 14200, Geschäftsführer Björn Nolting — 7

Identifikation: **Horse:** , **Color:** , **Breed:** , **Gender:** , **DOB.:** , **Registration N**

Eyes: Signs of disease of the conjunctiva, Cornea, anterior chamber, iris, lens, vitreous body,

Retina: ☐ no ____________________

Peripheral nervous system: ☐ normal ____________________

Oral cavity, Bite (visual inspection) ☐ normal ____________________

Ext. Reproductive organs (palpation and visual inspection): ☐ normal ____________________

Manure Quality: ☐ normal ____________________

Other: ____________________

B. II. Examination of the Legs and Feet

Manual inspection and Palpation of the legs: [e.g.: Conformation, Hoof shape and condition, Shoeing]

	Conformation from Front			Conformation from the side			Shoeing							Hoofs						Digital Tendon Sheath				
	Normal	Base Narrow	Base Wide	Normal	Over at the	Back at the knees	Normal	No Shoes	Overdue	Degree Pad	Too tight/ small	Plate	Other	Normal	Steep angle	Flat angle	Too	Very wide	Hoofwall flaky	Normal	Filled	Very filled	Hardened	Painful
Left Front																								
Right Front																								
Left Hind																								
Right Hind																								

Other:

Left front: ____________________

Right front: ____________________

Left hind: ____________________

Right hind: ____________________

Palpation of the back: ☐ normal

____

3. Evaluation at a Walk and Trot (Horse being led) – Straight Line/Circle - Hard Ground

☐ normal ____________________

4. Indications of ataxia: ☐ no ____________________

5. Inducible Pain:

a) Painful when turning: ☐ no ____________________

b) Flexion Test of the Legs:

Flexion Test:			**Trot after 1 Min. flexion**					**Explanation:**
Left front :	☐ no	☐ yes	LF:	-	±	+	++	- : clear Trot
Right front:	☐ no	☐ yes	RF:	-	±	+	++	± : first 3 steps questionable
Left hind:	☐ no	☐ yes	LH:	-	±	+	++	+ : ca. 10 steps lame
Right hind:	☐ no	☐ yes	RH:	-	±	+	++	++: lame

Tierärztliche Praxis für
Dr. Björn Nolting GmbH

Sitz: Weilerswist

Amtsgericht Bonn HRB 14200
Geschäftsführer Björn Nolting

8

Identifikation: Horse: , Color: , Breed: , Gender: , DOB.: , Registration No.:

B.III. EXAMINATION OF THE HEART, RESPIRATORY SYSTEM AND MOTION APPARATUS WHILE EXERCISED (EXERCISED UNTIL BREATHING LABORED) ☐ longed ☐ ridden

1. Abnormal breathing sounds: ☐ no ☐ on inspiration ☐ on expiration
2. Problems breathing: ☐ no ______
3. Problems moving: ☐ no ______
4. Coughing, Nasal discharge: ☐ no ______
5. Auscultation: Heart: ☐ normal ______
   Lung: ☐ normal ______
6. Pulse and Respiratory Rate :
   AFTER EXERCISING IN A ☐ Trot ☐ Canter

	BEFORE EXERCISE	AFTER EXERCISE	RECOVERY TIME
Pulse Rate			
Respiratory Rate			

B. IV. SPECIAL EXAMINATIONS:

I. Radiological Examination : ☐ radiographed ☐ not radiographed

1. Lateral view of the lower left front leg (Overview of the latero-medial view of the hoof, pastern joint, fetlock joint and sesamoid bones): ☐ not radiographed ☐ normal
   Findings: ______
2. Lateral view of the lower right front leg (Overview of the latero-medial view of the hoof, pastern joint, fetlock joint and sesamoid bones) ☐ not radiographed ☐ normal
   Findings: ______
3. Lateral view of the lower left hind leg (Overview of the latero-medial view of the hoof, pastern joint, fetlock joint and sesamoid bones): ☐ not radiographed ☐ normal
   Findings: ______
4. Lateral view of the lower right hind leg (Overview of the latero-medial view of the hoof, pastern joint, fetlock joint and sesamoid bones): ☐ not radiographed ☐ normal
   Findings: ______
5. A 45° view of the navicular bone "Oxspring" left front (dorso-palmar view of the navicular bone): ☐ not radiographed ☐ normal
   Findings: ______
6. A 45° view of the navicular bone "Oxspring" right front (dorso-palmar view of the navicular bone): ☐ not radiographed ☐ normal
   Findings: ______
7. Oblique view of the left hock approx. 90-115°: ☐ not radiographed ☐ normal
   Findings: ______
8. Oblique view of the left hock approx. 45-70°: ☐ not radiographed ☐ normal
   Findings: ______
9. Oblique view of the right hock approx. 90-115°: ☐ not radiographed ☐ normal
   Findings: ______
10. Oblique view of the right hock approx. 45-70°: ☐ not radiographed ☐ normal
    Findings: ______

Tierärztliche Praxis für Dr. Björn Nolting GmbH   Sitz: Weilerswist   Amtsgericht Bonn HRB 14200 Geschäftsführer Björn Nolting   9

Identifikation: **Horse: , Color: , Breed: , Gender: , DOB.: , Registration No.:**

11. Right hock (0°-dorso-plantar view):
☐ not radiographed ☐ normal
Findings: ______________________________

12. Left hock (0°-dorso-plantar view):
☐ not radiographed ☐ normal
Findings: ______________________________

b) additional views:

13. Left stifle (latero-medial view of the patella and parts of femur & tibia):
☐ not radiographed ☐ normal
Findings: ______________________________

14. Right stifle (latero-medial view of the patella and parts of femur & tibia)
☐ not radiographed ☐ normal
Findings: ______________________________

15. Dorsal spinous processes (End of withers/saddle area/lumbar area):
☐ not radiographed ☐ normal
Findings: ______________________________

16. Skyline view of the left front navicular bone (flexor surface view of the navicular bone):
☐ not radiographed ☐ normal
Findings: ______________________________

17. Skyline view of the left front navicular bone (flexor surface view of the navicular bone):
☐ not radiographed ☐ normal
Findings: ______________________________

Other Radiographs :

____

____

____

____

II. Endoscopy of the upper Airways:

☐ not performed ☐ normal ☐ Printed Pictures ☐ Sedated

____

____

____

III. Other Examinations:

____

____

____

IV. Drug Test:

☐ Blood not taken ☐ blood taken and examined ☐ blood taken and frozen (stored for 6 months)

Tierärztliche Praxis für
Dr. Björn Nolting GmbH

Sitz: Weilerswist

Amtsgericht Bonn HRB 14200
Geschäftsführer Björn Nolting

10

Identifikation: Horse: , Color: , Breed: , Gender: , DOB.: , Registration No.:

C. EVALUATION OF THE EXAMINATION RESULTS:

THE ABNORMAL BEHAVIOUR CRIBBING & WEAVING COULD NOT BE TESTED!

- ☐ The declaration to be made by the seller or his/her representative (see B.1 History: Declaration by seller/representative) was not completed. This lack of past information (health, vaccination and performance status) may lead to misinterpretation of examination results by the examining veterinarian or to miss abnormalities (surgical scars, behavioural problems, allergies).
- ☐ Todays examination does not indicate the existence of significant health problems.

THE CUSTOMER OR REPRESENTATIVE CONFIRMS THAT THE CONTRACT IS PART OF THE PRE-PURCHASE EXAMINATION AND THAT HE/SHE HAS BEEN INFORMED ABOUT ANY POTENTIAL RISKS ASSOCIATED WITH THE FINDING OF PROBLEMS IDENTIFIED BY THE VETERINARIAN. THE PERSON SIGNING THIS DOCUMENT EXPRESSIVELY CONFIRMS THAT HE/SHE IS AUTHORIZED TO MAKE ALL STATEMENTS NECESSARY DURING THE PRE-PURCHASE EXAM CONCERNING THIS HORSE AND ALSO BE THE RECIPIENT OF THE EXPLANATION OF THE EXAMINATION RESULTS. HE/SHE ALSO CONFIRMS THE VALUE/PRICE OF THE HORSE AS STATED IN § 6 & § 7 OF THIS CONTRACT. THE SHORTENED STATUTE OF LIMITATIONS TO SIX MONTHS IS MADE KNOWINGLY AND IS HEREBY CONFIRMED.

________________,the______________ X____________________

Place Date Client or Representative

____________________ ____________________

Other persons present Examining Veterinarian

Tierärztliche Praxis für Dr. Björn Nolting GmbH Sitz: Weilerswist Amtsgericht Bonn HRB 14200 Geschäftsführer Björn Nolting 11